T0209011

THE
UTERINE
HEALTH
COMPANION

THE
UTERINE
HEALTH
COMPANION

A HOLISTIC GUIDE TO LIFELONG WELLNESS

Eve Agee, PhD

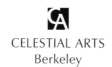

CELESTIAL ARTS
Berkeley

Disclaimer: The information contained in this book is based on the experience and research of the author. It is not intended as a substitute for consulting with your physician or other health care provider. Any attempt to diagnose and treat an illness should be done under the direction of a health care professional. The publisher and author are not responsible for any adverse effects or consequences resulting from the use of any of the suggestions, preparations, or procedures discussed in this book.

Copyright © 2010 by Eve Agee

All rights reserved.
Published in the United States by Celestial Arts, an imprint of the
Crown Publishing Group, a division of Random House, Inc., New York.
www.crownpublishing.com
www.tenspeed.com

Celestial Arts and the Celestial Arts colophon are registered trademarks
of Random House, Inc.

Library of Congress Cataloging-in-Publication Data
Agee, Eve.
  The uterine health companion : a holistic guide to lifelong wellness / Eve Agee.
     p. cm.
  Summary: "For women interested in a holistic approach to maintaining
optimal uterine health and addressing specific health disorders of the
uterus, from menarche to menopause and beyond"—Provided by publisher.
  Includes bibliographical references and index.
  1. Uterus—Diseases—Alternative treatment. 2. Holistic medicine. 3. Women—Health
and hygiene. I. Title.
  RG301.A35 2010
  618.1'4—dc22
  2009040100

ISBN 978-1-58761-351-7

Design by Chloe Rawlins

First Edition

146119709

Contents

To women everywhere.
May your creative power shine freely.

Acknowledgments

I feel deeply blessed that this book has been helped along the way by so many brilliant and generous souls. I am deeply grateful to all the women and health care providers in the United States and West Africa who so graciously participated in my anthropology research and shared their wisdom and insights with me. I am truly appreciative of my wonderful clients with whom it has been an honor to work.

Special thanks go to Dr. David Buckley and Dr. Kim Agee for their careful reading of the medical sections of each chapter and their willingness to answer my questions. I extend my deepest appreciation to nutritionist Catherine Varchaver for her thorough review and suggestions for the nutrition chapter and naturopath Jennifer Neill for her recommendations regarding herbs, supplements, nutrition, and postural awareness. I am grateful to acupuncturist Diane Shandor and reflexologist Sally Wimberly for their contributions to this book. I send gratitude to my coaching and holistic health teachers and colleagues, especially Ken and Renee Kizer, Robert Warwick, and Ti Caine.

Many thanks go to my University of Virginia friends and colleagues who supported me during the first stages of research and writing, including Dr. Edy Gonzalez de Scollard, Sarah Boone, Dr. Anjana Mebane Cruz, Drake Patten, Hank Lewis, Drs. Eleanor and Tom Nevins, and Dr. Dan Friedman. I am also grateful to Dr. Gertrude Fraser, Dr. Susan McKinnon,

Dr. George Mentore, and Dr. Roy Wagner for their anthropological exper-tise and mentoring.

I want to express heartfelt thanks to all of my amazing friends, espe-cially to those who have given time and energy to help this book be born, including Danny Maiello, Vivian Schilling, Eric Parkinson, Kendall Helm, Rose Bunch, Chad Taylor, and Melodie Tsai. I extend a special acknowledgment to Pam Marraccini for her invaluable partnership in earlier phases of this project.

My sincere gratitude goes to all the talented people at Celestial Arts/ Ten Speed Press. I am so grateful for my magnificent editor, Sara Golski. This book has been vastly enriched by her remarkable clarity and aware-ness. I also want to thank Genoveva Llosa and Kristi Hein for their con-tributions. I am profoundly grateful to my extraordinary agents, Howard Yoon and Gail Ross, for their skill, commitment, and vision.

I would like to acknowledge my entire extended family for their love and encouragement. My deepest thanks go to my husband, Scott, for his ongoing understanding and belief in my work. I am also thankful to my son, Xavier, for all the exuberance, inspiration, and playfulness that he brings into my life. I extend immense gratitude to my mother, Martha; my late father, Jake; my sisters, Chandra and Mignonne; and my brother, Kim, for their lifelong support. I am truly grateful to my late grandparents, Lottie McCracken, Russell McCracken, Ora Agee, and Asa Agee, and to all my ancestors and guides for the gifts they have given me. I want to especially acknowledge my great-aunt Elsie McCracken for teaching me about holistic health traditions during my childhood. Finally, I thank the divine universe for the guidance, energy, and opportunity to bring this book into being.

Introduction:
Celebrating the Uterus

The drumbeat sent waves of pleasure to my heart as the air filled with the smell of fry bread cooking on an outdoor grill. The two young women dancing in front of me had not eaten since before sunrise, yet they moved with grace and ease. Sweat started to drip down their beautiful faces now that the luminous morning sun had finally emerged to begin shining on this ceremony.

In the vast field where the extraordinary rite occurred, the two teenage girls were the center of attention. They were surrounded by a crowd of friends, family, and other tribal members who would help them keep the beat of the drums for much of the next few days. They joyfully danced together on the hard Arizona ground for hours at a time.

It was 1999, and I had traveled to the White Mountain Apache tribal lands to witness the Sunrise Ceremony commemorating the beginning of two young women's menstrual cycles. An anthropologist colleague who knew of my work in women's health invited me to this age-old ritual that marks a girl's passage into womanhood. It is the most celebrated event in Apache culture.

For five days, I was riveted as the reservation filled with dancers, drummers, and hundreds of men and women who came from throughout New Mexico and Arizona to pay tribute to these two teenagers, Nashota and Zaltana,[1] who embarked on menarche within months of each other the previous year. People chanted and danced under the hot Arizona sun to honor these young women for starting their periods.

During the ceremony, Zaltana and Nashota ascended to almost divine status as they embodied the Apache goddess, Changing Woman. The young women laid their hands on the other participants, bestowing curative energy to their tribe. The ritual culminated with the exchange of truckloads of gifts to inaugurate Nashota's and Zaltana's relationships with their new godmothers, who would help guide them into adulthood.

During my time there, Apache men and women spoke to me about the power of women and menstruation to transform, heal, and purify. They were perplexed by white people's views of the menstrual cycle. Most Native Americans consider menstruation, pregnancy, and meno-pause as life-affirming processes that connect women to the earth, the moon, and the cycles of nature. I realized that this celebration was just the beginning of a beautiful relationship with menstruation for Nashota and Zaltana. They were poised to have a whole lifetime of feeling posi-tive about their periods.

After I left the reservation, I couldn't help thinking what would it be like for the rest of us if our cultures congratulated us on menarche and believed that women became powerful by menstruating—rather than fre-quently disparaging women as emotionally unstable during our periods. On a deeper level, I wondered how it would affect our lives if we as women felt good about our menstrual cycles and menopause transitions and looked forward to the cyclical changes in our bodies. Would we still have such severe aches, pain, and mood swings, or would our discomfort and anger melt in the face of deep respect and awe of our uterine processes?

In contrast to the Apache custom of celebrating every girl's men-arche, Julia, a seventeen-year-old white American I interviewed a few years later, shared that she did not even tell her mother when she first begin menstruating at age twelve. In a hushed voice, she revealed to me that embarrassment compelled her to hide the fact from her mother. Julia smiled wryly as she told me that she figured out how to use tam-pons from the pamphlet in the box. Her mother found out what had happened only when she started her own period a little later that month and noticed that the tampons were nearly gone. Julia became slightly fidgety as she described her feelings when her mother confronted her. "I felt ashamed when she came and asked me [if I had started]. She said it was no big deal, but I still don't like anyone else to know when it is going on."

Sacred Processes

Beyond the familiar cloak of silence that Julia describes exists a world where uterine processes are revered and celebrated. The Apache understanding of menstruation may seem foreign to you and me. However, there are millions of people throughout the planet who consider menstruation and menopause beneficial—even sacred. We most frequently find these cultural attitudes in indigenous and polytheist societies in Africa, Asia, and the Americas that honor the feminine as part of the divine.

There are, of course, non-Western societies that view women's bodies and uterine processes negatively, most frequently those that worship a monotheistic male divinity, such as Christianity, Islam, and Judiasm. We witness these attitudes carried out through work, sex, and religious restrictions on menstruating and menopausal women, and to the extreme in the tragic practice of female genital mutilation. Even in cultures that do not necessarily hold negative views about uterine processes, menstruation can sometimes pose obstacles to women and girls—especially as indigenous societies adopt Western practices. For example, girls in some parts of Africa cannot attend school while menstruating because of the lack of feminine hygiene products, running water, and bathroom facilities.

However, there are many contemporary cultures that regard menopause and menstruation as positive and support women during their uterine processes—even though we rarely hear about them in the news. I was first exposed to this affirming viewpoint while living in West Africa in the early 1990s. While conducting medical anthropology research, I observed that Mossi women in Burkina Faso take time away from their work and cooking for their families for the length of every menstrual period to enjoy creative endeavors or visit with friends. Also in West Africa, the Dagara ethnic group believes that menstruating women possess heightened wisdom and healing power. The Mbuti pygmies of Central Africa regard menstrual blood as a gift that is honored by their whole community.

In parts of Southern India, newly menstruating girls are given feasts, money, and gifts and are adorned in beautiful new clothes. Japanese families traditionally commemorate a daughter's first menstrual period by eating red rice and beans. Aboriginal Australians ritually bathe and apply beautiful body paint to young women at the onset of their periods. Many Native American tribes believe that menstruation naturally cleanses women so they do not need to detoxify in ritual sweat lodges as men do.

Indigenous people throughout the planet view menopausal women as wise women and leaders. In West Africa, I found that menopause is considered a gift to Togolese women healers, who use the extra body heat that some women experience during the transformation to heal others and master their craft. Many Native Americans believe that the menopausal process enhances visionary abilities, foresight, and wisdom. In Thailand, women describe looking forward to menopause and the increased status it gives them.

Strikingly, these cross-cultural differences extend well beyond attitudes. Women in non-Western and indigenous societies rarely share in the high rates of benign uterine health problems experienced by Western women. Many African women do not experience PMS or problems with menstruation. Indigenous women interviewed in Latin America reported no negative physical side effects from menopause. Medical anthropology researchers in Japan found that there was no equivalent word for "hot flash" in Japanese. Twelve percent of the women in their study recounted occasionally being hotter than usual, but did not attribute their experiences to menopause or feel that it was particularly problematic.[2]

A Western Health Crisis

Yet every day, millions of women in the Western world face debilitating uterine health disorders. Millions of American women experience PMS or painful menstruation. More than four million American women have endometriosis, a condition in which the uterine lining grows outside of the uterus, causing severe menstrual pain and frequent infertility. Twenty-five percent of women in the United States report pain from uterine fibroids each year, and as many as 75 percent may have fibroids. Nearly 30 percent of all pregnancies end in miscarriage, and more than three million women encounter infertility problems. The numbers don't stop here.

Every hour, seventy-two American women have hysterectomies, the highest rate in the world. Hysterectomy is the surgical removal of the uterus, after which women cannot have children. In total, twelve million of our neighbors, sisters, colleagues, mothers, and friends have had hysterectomies during the past twenty years. Millions more who have decided against this surgery have had to live with chronic pain and fatigue. By age sixty, one-third of all American women have had hysterectomies.

The numbers are just as startling across the Atlantic. In Europe, more than fourteen million women have endometriosis. Twenty-five percent have painful uterine fibroid tumors. Even down under in Australia, non-indigenous women have one of the highest rates of debilitating PMS in the world.

As these statistics suggest, there is a major uterine health crisis in Western countries, yet very few people in the medical field acknowledge it as such. Even though these benign uterine conditions are not life-threatening, they can have a devastating impact on women's lives. I first became aware of this unrecognized crisis as a medical anthropologist researching women's health during the late 1990s. I began my investigation to understand why American women have such high rates of menopausal problems and symptoms compared to women in other areas of the world, specifically Africa. As my research progressed and I realized that this pattern affected Western women of all ages, I decided to widen the scope of my study.

In my research, I observed more than four hundred consultations between doctors and female patients of varying ages concerning uterine health issues. For three years, I shadowed twenty doctors in four clinics in one of the top health care systems in the United States. I observed doctor-patient consultations and interviewed physicians, nurses, health educators, policy makers, and female patients about their interactions and the state of women's health. I have interviewed more than three hundred American women about their uterine health and the impact it has on their lives.

I was shocked by my findings. Large numbers of women—from their twenties to their seventies—had debilitating uterine health problems. High percentages of female patients reported uterine health problems such as fibroids, endometriosis, and PMS, as well as menopausal symptoms lasting more than a decade. Many of these women experienced heavy bleeding, exhaustion, and hot flashes that made it difficult to work, leave their homes, or get a good night's sleep. My heart opened up to these women: the very fabric of their lives was compromised, yet most seemed embarrassed to even talk to their physicians about their uterine problems.

Frustrated doctors would often tell me that beyond hysterectomy, there were not many avenues for permanently ceasing their patients' constant bleeding, pain, and fatigue, especially for those who wanted to have children. Several physicians expressed concern that more successful treatment options didn't exist. Pharmaceutical and other less-invasive treatments are available, but most have undesirable side effects or health risks, or do not provide effective long-term relief for many women. With conditions such as endometriosis and chronic pelvic pain, symptoms recur in one quarter of all cases even after the uterus has been surgically removed.

At night, as I sat at home to write my field notes, I was haunted by the images I witnessed in the hospitals and doctors' offices during the day. So many women in the most powerful society in the world were routinely suffering from extreme pain associated with their uteruses—a saddening fact. I couldn't believe that at the dawn of the twenty-first century, hysterectomy was still being used as one the main forms of treatment for a wide variety of uterine problems. In my research I met some women who got relief from their hysterectomies and just as many who experienced painful ongoing side effects from the surgery. I was troubled that preventative measures that would help women avoid benign uterine problems were not regularly discussed with most women and that there were so few effective alternatives for women who still wanted to get pregnant or simply not have part of their bodies removed.

Certainly, biomedicine has provided women with many important health advantages, such as technologies that have significantly lowered maternal death rates in the societies where high-tech birthing methods are available. Additionally, early detection methods developed in the 1970s have greatly reduced rates of cervical cancer in the United States and Europe compared to developing countries where women do not have regular access to Pap tests. However, since that time, nonmalignant uterine problems (the focus of this book) have remained high in the West—and have increased among young women in their teens and twenties.

I wondered why, thirty years after the women's health movement began, most of the cutting-edge technologies in uterine health centered around fertility and birth, whereas there were few successful advancements in other areas of uterine wellness that would guarantee all women better quality of life. I was outraged that biomedicine had come so far in its ability to heal the heart and many other complicated bodily systems, but seemed to lack similar research and development with uterine health and prevention that would allow women to keep their bodies healthy and intact.

The Stigma of the Uterus

As I deepened my research, I discovered that this lack of successful treatment options might stem in part from the very perception of the uterus in contemporary Western medicine and culture. Instead of dreading their menses, early humans cherished the uterus and women's cycles of menstruation, pregnancy, birth, and menopause. The uterus was considered sacred in much of early Africa, Asia, Native America, and Europe.

Many prehistoric societies celebrated the uterus as the body's center of female power and creativity. Numerous indigenous cultures believed that it was through the power of the uterus that the goddess gave birth to the world. Treasured and important, the uterus was historically painted and sculpted on the female form and portrayed in representations of women and goddesses throughout Europe and Asia. Drawings of the uterus have been found on cave walls, elaborate tombs and drums, as well as shrines honoring the divine feminine. The remains of these cultures reveal that societal respect and awe of the uterus existed across much of early Europe, Asia, Africa, and the Americas.

However, as the basis of Western medicine was taking root, the view of women's bodies and power in ancient Greece shifted. At the birth of biomedicine, the uterus came to be considered a polluting factor for women's health. The first physicians deemed the uterus unstable, citing it as the reason behind insanity or instability in their female patients. In fact, "hysteria" (derived from *hyster*, the Greek term for uterus) was considered a condition in which a woman's insanity was caused by her uterus.

In more recent eras, Victorian doctors believed that removing the female organs would allow women and girls to gain mental stability and become better wives. Surgeries such as hysterectomies, clitoridectomies, and oophorectomies (removal of the ovaries) were employed in poorly executed attempts to "heal" kleptomania, epilepsy, melancholy, and hysteria in the United States and England. By the 1930s, clitoridectomies ceased to be performed in mental hospitals in the United States. Yet well into the 1950s, hysterectomies continued to be used in misguided efforts to improve the quality of women's lives—even in cases in which there was nothing medically wrong with the patient's uterus.

Thankfully, we no longer follow these archaic practices in North America and Europe. However, as Westerners, most of us still consider the uterus naturally problematic. Many of us *expect* women to have problems with menstruation, birth, and menopause. We frequently assume cyclical pain and suffering are an inherent and unavoidable part of being a woman.

Perhaps unsurprisingly, I regularly saw these attitudes about uterine health reflected in my research with contemporary doctors. When I mentioned my concerns about the high rates of PMS, fibroids, endometriosis, pelvic pain, and menopausal difficulties to the physicians and nurses with whom I worked, they assured me that these patterns of uterine dysfunction were the norm. For the most part, they explained that all they could do was help their patients manage their conditions with medication, hysterectomies, or less-invasive surgical procedures.

As a medical anthropologist, I looked at the situation through a different lens. I talked to doctors about finding new ways to reduce rates of chronic uterine ailments, but they seemed uninterested in the research from non-Western cultures that challenged such high rates of benign uterine disorders. Most physicians dismissed my questions about the efficacy of preventative care strategies for uterine wellness or suggested that most of their patients would not be willing or able to make major lifestyle changes as easily as they could take a pill. Some suggested that if a woman's health became bad enough she could just have a hysterectomy to make her problem go away.

Of course, I encountered some doctors who greatly enjoy preventative medicine and women's well care who do not like to perform hysterectomies until all other options have been ruled out. Many are gynecologists who have a strong passion for women's health or family practice doctors who tend to regularly focus on lifelong prevention with their patients. One specialty menopause clinic where I did my observations had a health educator who counseled patients on using nutrition and stress reduction to reduce symptoms. Even though the American College of Obstetricians and Gynecologists includes nutrition, exercise, and stress reduction guidelines for reducing PMS, menstrual pain, and menopause symptoms, the majority of gynecologists in my study expressed sincere enthusiasm for surgery and delivering babies—and skepticism toward lifestyle approaches for preventing benign uterine problems.

Like the rest of our society, medical researchers and physicians have been indoctrinated to see uterine problems as natural or perhaps inevitable. From this view, our current uterine health crisis simply looks the way we have all been conditioned to think women's health is meant to be—inconvenient, painful, or embarrassing. We lack the passion that would spark research and technology to bring about a cure, because of the negative perspective that we in the West have of the uterus.

Our cultural blinders create shame that makes some physicians, researchers, drug companies, and women want to sweep nonreproductive uterine processes under the proverbial rug. Consequently, technologies focus on helping the uterus disappear, through either pharmaceutical treatments that erase all traces of our natural processes (making menstruating women no longer bleed and menopausal women menstruate) or surgeries that simply get rid of the uterus. Preventative strategies that are widely promoted in many other areas of health for men and women are not discussed as frequently as treatment options for uterine problems, even though research shows that nutrition, stress reduction, and other lifestyle changes can be profoundly effective for establishing uterine wellness.

Another Way

The personal implications of my research inspired me to look beyond Western medicine, to find more low-risk strategies for preventing non-cancerous uterine problems, such as PMS, fibroid tumors, endometriosis, or menopausal symptoms. I researched other healing systems to see whether they offered any avenues for creating uterine wellness and preventing disease with fewer side effects. Expanding my horizons to include mind-body medicine revealed many effective strategies as well as affirming viewpoints about the significance of the uterus in women's health.

Scientific research shows that multiple complementary medicine traditions provide nervous system support, hormonal balancing, and stress reduction, all of which can offer significant protection against and relief for uterine disorders. Acupuncture relieves pain and symptoms related to PMS, menopause, pregnancy, and birth, and it can assist with some types of fertility treatments. Chiropractic treatments can reduce menstrual and menopausal problems and strengthen the nervous system to help ease endometriosis and fibroid pain. Both acupuncture and chiropractic treatments can correct fetal positioning during the third trimester to aid with birth. Many women also report that massage and other types of bodywork promote increased uterine wellness and decreased pain.

Energy modalities such as acupuncture, Reiki, and Healing Touch are increasingly used in hospitals to lessen pain and accelerate recovery from surgery and chemotherapy. Acupressure also alleviates pain, nausea, and vomiting after gynecological surgery while avoiding the side effects of medication.

Most mind-body healing traditions offer effective self-care techniques women can integrate into their lives to create uterine wellness. Practices such as relaxation and cognitive restructuring can cut PMS symptoms in half. A 2005 report in the *Journal of the American Medical Association* confirms that stress-reducing lifestyle changes, such as practicing yoga or improving dietary intake, helped menopausal women achieve more long-lasting symptom relief than hormone therapy, which lost its efficacy as soon as the medication was discontinued.[3] Visualization and guided imagery techniques have been proven to decrease pain in many studies and are effective with diminishing pain from PMS, fibroids, menopause, and endometriosis.

Integrative nutrition has been demonstrated to significantly improve endometriosis, PMS, menopausal symptoms, and uterine pain. Without proper diet and the absorption of essential nutrients, hormones become imbalanced, affecting the endocrine glands, uterus, and ovaries. The high prevalence of estrogen in the typical Western diet exacerbates uterine problems. Women can promote uterine wellness and prevent inflammation by increasing their intake of vegetables, fruits, healthy oils, and whole grains while decreasing their consumption of animal protein, sugar, and refined foods.

Herbs have been used to support uterine processes in cultures throughout the world. Recent research reveals that this age-old practice can help many uterine conditions. Red raspberry, black cohosh, dong quai, and wild yam assist in maintaining or restoring menstrual, pregnancy, and menopausal wellness. Additionally, turmeric, ginger, and burdock root may ameliorate fibroid symptoms.

In addition to their efficacy in preventing and healing uterine imbalances, many mind-body healing systems offer empowering ways of viewing the uterus. These traditions reflect the cultures from which they originate, many of which share positive perspectives on uterine health. In most holistic medical frameworks, the uterus is an integral part of women's health.

My quest to find successful noninvasive uterine health care options led me to my career as a healer and life coach specializing in women's wellness and empowerment. In my work with clients, I have seen first-hand how mind-body modalities can complement our current medical model. These practices help us take a more holistic approach to women's health instead of narrowly focusing on individual problems of the uterus without understanding how they relate to previous uterine imbalances or other aspects of women's lives.

Women can use complementary techniques to heal their bodies, their beliefs, and any facets of their lives that are out of balance, to move beyond symptom management and achieve lifelong wellness. You can implement measures to attend to your uterine health in the same way you take preventative actions to take care of your heart, bones, and teeth. Mind-body techniques can help you enhance the efficacy of standard biomedical treatments and prevent future uterine imbalances from occurring. Opening up to holistic approaches can also assist you in developing more positive attitudes about uterine health.

This book is full of integrative strategies you can use to create uterine wellness. Chapters one and two discuss the cornerstones of holistic health and the importance of the uterus to our whole body health. Chapters three through five outline my holistic plan—the Optimal Uterine Health Plan—involving conscious breathing, visualization, stress reduction, nutrition, exercise, postural alignment, and other mind-body healing for achieving optimal uterine health. Chapters six through eleven provide methods to help heal and prevent specific uterine conditions. The conclusion proposes increasing public outreach so that all women know that the uterus is worth taking care of. It also discusses ways we can more fully appreciate our uterine processes and celebrate our lives as powerful, creative women.

My suggestions focus on self-care treatments you can perform at home and combine easily with standard biomedical care. You may wish to seek additional assistance from an acupuncturist, naturopath, chiropractor, integrative nutritionist, massage therapist, breathing coach, or other mind-body therapist if you feel it will enhance your health. I fully encourage you to discuss all complementary therapies with your doctor.

It is my honor to share this story of women's courage and new possibilities with you. Entering this world of holistic healing dramatically transformed my own life. I hope it will enrich your relationship with your body and create waves of change that will improve women's health in our country and in the world.

PART ONE

Understanding Uterine Health

CHAPTER ONE

Holistic Health Foundations

As a young girl, you might have giggled, squirmed, or looked away as you learned about the female reproductive system in school. Many of our mothers rarely shared much additional knowledge about "what goes on down there" except to tell us how to stay clean and not get pregnant. This incomplete introduction to the uterus epitomizes most Western women's relationship to this purely female organ. Forgotten, cursed, or ignored, our uteruses are considered by most of us to be either problematic or insignificant—except on the occasions we focus our attention on becoming pregnant.

However, for every human being, the uterus is our first home. It is our original source of life as humans and, at least so far, essential to our continuance as a race. You and I both began in a uterus and so did everyone else we know.

In my mid-twenties, it was my interest in our society's attitudes about the uterus that kept me home in the United States to study menopause instead of going to West Africa as I had originally planned. At the time, I was a doctoral student in anthropology at the University of Virginia. I was intrigued with the then-blossoming field of medical anthropology and knew I wanted to study women's health as an anthropologist.

I had previously lived, studied, and taught in the small West African country of Togo. When I began grad school, I assumed I would move to Togo for several years to conduct my dissertation research, a traditional anthropology rite of passage. However, political conditions in Togo had exploded, making it no longer a viable option. While doing anthropological research in the neighboring country of Burkina Faso, I learned more about the divergence of uterine health patterns between American and African women. I discovered that some West African women looked positively on menstruation and menopause, which made me wonder why our society approached these same bodily processes with such embarrassment and apprehension. I felt that I needed to understand my own culture's gender attitudes and experiences before continuing my research elsewhere.

I decided to follow in the footsteps of some of the most cutting-edge ethnographic research at the time, which involved turning the cultural microscope on ourselves to better understand the patterns influencing our lives and health care. I chose to stay in the States and focus my investigation on African-American and white women to explore how race and class affect women's attitudes and experiences with their health. I conducted a portion of my study in clinical settings to learn more about the ways in which women are treated in our health care system.

When I begin my fieldwork, I was not certain that I would have as much access to my research subjects' lives as I was honored to have as an anthropologist in Africa. To my surprise, the people in my study graciously welcomed me into their work and their lives. Doctors, nurses, and health educators let me observe their interactions with their patients. These health care providers took the time to talk to me about their hopes, concerns, and grievances about their careers. Women invited me into their homes or met me for interviews, where they shared intimate pictures of the ways their uterine health impacted their lives and bodies. During interviews, women frequently told me I was the first person other than their doctors with whom they had spoken so candidly about these issues. A few women expressed embarrassment in talking about their uterine health. Several women told me that they were so reluctant to talk about menstruation that they generally put off visiting their doctors about excessive bleeding or painful periods until their situation was so debilitating that they had to seek help. However, the majority seemed to enjoy being freely able to discuss their experiences with someone who was truly interested.

Hundreds of women kindly allowed me into the treatment rooms where they experienced the vulnerability inherent to gynecological exams. They let me be present while they were diagnosed with fibroids, endometriosis, early menopause, and cancer, or were presented with the treatment options available for their conditions. I attended support groups for perimenopausal and menopausal women looking for assistance for conditions that many thought were too taboo to discuss openly with friends and family.

A Researcher's Journey

My investigation of uterine health connected me to my roots in a surprising way. I was raised in an environment that revered medical science. My father was a dentist, and other family members and friends were dentists or physicians. I had pondered becoming a physician myself and considered getting a dual PhD/MD focusing on women's health—until my research took me down an unexpected path.

I grew up in the Arkansas Ozarks, where holistic health modalities were practiced widely until my parents' generation. My maternal grandparents and great-aunt had been raised using these complementary techniques. They all had advanced college degrees, and my great-aunt was a certified reflexologist and nutritionist. My grandmother was a university professor, while my grandfather was a school superintendent and principal. They used biomedicine as their primary form of health care, yet they integrated nutrition and reflexology into their self-care. When I was young, they taught me about reflexology, herbs, crystals, and organic farming. My great-aunt encouraged me and my siblings to study holistic health and other cultural traditions.

My father and his colleagues embraced biomedicine as the way of the future. They regarded these mind-body health customs as antiquated and outdated, and they instilled in me a view of medical science as the only way of tending to my health. My father and siblings laughed at my mother's family's "weird habits." By ten or eleven, I too began to brush off this traditional knowledge. As a teenager, I ignored my grandparents' and great-aunt's suggestions on how I could use holistic methods to improve my health. However, when my research began to reveal that, at least in the area of women's health, Western medicine did not have all the answers, I realized that perhaps the elders in my family had been onto something after all.

Shortly after I started my research, a twist of fate reintroduced me to holistic medicine at a time when I was ready to listen and learn. A native healer I met through a common friend suggested that she could teach me about mind-body approaches. I began apprenticing with this practitioner, who combined Cherokee therapies from her family background with Asian and African mind-body techniques. For more than three years, I studied visualization, meditation, guided imagery, energetic balancing, herbs, and intuitive healing under her guidance.

By the time I completed my PhD, I knew I wanted to help bring this information about the power of complementary medicine to the world, so I continued to look for opportunities that would help increase my knowledge. I moved to Washington, D.C. where I worked as a political appointee in the administration of President Bill Clinton and continued my integrative health training.

In the Clinton administration, I worked with the White House, Congress, and other federal agencies to improve the educational and health opportunities for women and children. The experience opened my eyes to the ways government programs can assist people in creating better lives. It also helped me understand firsthand how corporate interests affect health care policies and practices, often to the detriment of our health and wellness. Even though this work was rewarding, I knew my purpose lay down a different road. I broadened my foundation in traditional healing by studying with a naturopath in Chicago and training in spiritual life coaching and conscious connected breathing facilitation in Maryland and Virginia.

I also expanded my anthropology research in women's health to other areas of the country. I interviewed more than one hundred white, African-American, Asian, Latina, and Native American women of all ages throughout the United States. Like the women in the earlier phase of study, they generously disclosed their experiences and attitudes about uterine health to me. Additionally, I interviewed a cross-section of holistic healers to understand how different types of mind-body disciplines approach uterine health imbalances.

When the Clinton administration ended, I began my practice as a mind-body healer and life coach in Washington, D.C. My personal experience with an early miscarriage two years later motivated me to learn even more about using mind-body techniques to establish uterine wellness. During my subsequent pregnancy I delved deeper into holistic health traditions to help carry my pregnancy to term and experience natural childbirth.

I began to share this knowledge through workshops and private consultations, where I met hundreds of women with diverse uterine issues looking for effective noninvasive treatments. Integrating the expertise I acquired in the various branches of complementary medicine, I developed a program of nutritional support, stress reduction, life coaching, visualization, and transformational breathing that has assisted my clients in healing PMS, pelvic pain, infertility, menopausal symptoms, and other chronic health problems. Part two of this book, the Optimal Uterine Health Plan, grew out of this program for my clients.

In 2006, I returned to my hometown of Fayetteville, Arkansas, where I continue to assist women across the country and internationally with their healing and empowerment. Drawing on the experiences of my own clients as well as those of women who have healed their uterine problems using other complementary modalities—such as acupuncture, chiropractic medicine, nutrition, massage, and bodywork—I have written this book to help answer the urgent call for a healthier, whole-body approach to reducing uterine pain and problems.

The New Medicine

In *Visions: How Science Will Revolutionize the Twenty-First Century*, best-selling author and physicist Michio Kaku affirms that as more studies are done to demonstrate the immense effect of the mind-body connection on the cellular and molecular levels, medicine as we know it will be vastly improved.[1] Currently, biomedical treatments tend to isolate uterine dysfunctions without generally exploring women's nutritional, emotional, and exercise patterns—even though research shows that stress, lifestyle, and other mind-body factors have a huge impact on uterine health. This compartmentalized strategy is standard in our current health care system, because our entire scientific framework has been shaped by a four-hundred-year-old pact that physicians entered into in an effort to appease religious leaders. René Descartes, a seventeenth-century scientist and philosopher, made an agreement with the pope in order to be permitted to dissect human corpses. Descartes vowed that medicine would rule over only the physical body while leaving the mind, emotions, and spirit to the Church.

The Cartesian split continues to dominate medicine and science to this day. It has also encouraged our society to separate human experience into two distinct spheres: body and mind. This ideology positioned the body as a grouping of mechanical parts to be controlled by the mind rather than viewing human experience as a dynamic combination of body, mind, spirit, energy, and emotion, as holistic approaches do. In this process the rational intelligence of the mind (which Western culture associates with men) became elevated over embodied experience and knowledge, which have been considered the domain of women and female healers. This philosophy not only affects the way Western medicine is practiced, but also significantly influences the way you and I live and relate to our bodies.

The reintroduction of traditional medicine to the West in the past forty years, along with the findings of modern science, have challenged this mind-body separation. Non-Western medical systems have brought to light the importance of incorporating emotional, energetic, and societal factors on uterine wellness. In traditional Chinese medicine, for example, the uterus sits in the *dantian*, the body's energetic center. Chinese medicine proposes that there is an important relationship between the uterus and the heart, and biomedical research now confirms the influence of the uterus on heart health. The Chinese believe an energy channel runs though the core of every woman's torso connecting these two organs. Sadness, anger, and unresolved issues about one's relationships and identity as a woman move between the heart and the uterus, affecting women's cycles, reproductive health, and experiences during menopause. In this system, emotional healing is essential to strengthening uterine health.

In South Asian–based chakra healing, the uterus is situated in the second chakra, the body's center for creativity, relationships, sexuality, and financial prosperity. In this energy medicine system, the uterus embodies our capacity for relating to others as well as to the world at large. In the chakra framework, when our relationships and interactions are out of balance, the organs of the second chakra become weakened or diseased. If women continually block their personal power and creativity out of fear, the energy and health of the uterus will be negatively affected. Consequently, creative expression, healthy relationships, and opening up to personal power facilitate balanced energy and healing in the uterus.

Western medicine is at a crossroads where ineffective mechanistic practices are starting to be replaced by these and other integrative approaches. The emergence of holistic healing promises to revitalize a medical system that seems to be slowly running out of breath. Merging these methods will improve the efficacy and reduce the costs of our current medical system while bridging the expertise of so many talented biomedical and complementary practitioners. It will also help change Western medicine for the better by erasing the erroneous belief in a disconnection between body, mind, and spirit that has plagued our science and culture for the past four hundred years.

The most advanced levels of scientific research have heralded this new path, but putting research into practice is a slow process, especially in a world where medical practitioners are burdened by ever-expanding workloads and where funding for experiments is usually based on potential industry profits. At the top echelons of medical education, medical students are learning to embrace this innovative whole-body approach. I hold a vision that one day everyone will have access to quality health care that combines holistic methods with excellent biomedical care that focuses on keeping the whole person well. However, it may be many years before these new understandings trickle down to all medical specialties and practitioners. In the meantime, I encourage you to take your health into your own hands. As you learn to combine these two forms of medicine in the ways that work best for your own life, you will reap the health benefits that all of us deserve.

Shifting Fundamentals

As Westerners, most of us still give preference to our minds and thoughts, which we unsuccessfully use to attempt to control our emotions, energy, spirit, and bodies. One of the primary principles of mind-body healing involves letting go of this illusion of control and becoming conscious of your whole being. Most integrative approaches use the breath to assist people in connecting more deeply with body and spirit. I became aware of the power of the breath when I first lived in West Africa. I was nineteen when I left Arkansas and went to Togo, West Africa, to study French and learn about African culture. While I was there I knew that there was something very appealing about the Togolese that I could never quite put into words.

Even though most Togolese live on less than a dollar a day and face many other challenges far greater than most people face in the States, I rarely discerned the same levels of anxiety in Togo that we Americans experience frequently (even when our basic survival is in no way threatened). When I came back to the United States, I longed for that unnamed quality I had witnessed. As I progressed in my holistic health training, I realized that the energy I felt there was due in part to the Togolese tendencies to breathe deeply and fully inhabit their bodies.

I remembered seeing the breath moving through people's backs as they walked, worked, and carried on their daily lives. In a place where people's everyday struggles greatly outnumber ours, the cultural practice of deep breathing created a groundedness that I had rarely experienced in my life in the States. Through my studies I learned that deep breathing helps people balance their awareness evenly throughout their entire bodies rather than focusing their attention mainly on their thoughts and minds.

The simple act of deepening your breath will help you open up to the rich inner knowledge that is inside of you. Through conscious breathing, you can begin to recognize and release distracting chatter in your head and connect with the energy located in your body and spirit. Just as it is vital to have effective communication with your health care providers, mind-body traditions teach us that it is of equal or greater importance to have clear communication with your body and your inner guidance. Nobody knows your body better than you. However, the majority of us have been taught to ignore our own inner guidance and body knowledge and hand over our authority to people and institutions outside of ourselves such as our families, schools, the medical establishment, or the media.

In *The Woman in the Body*, anthropologist Emily Martin suggests that as women raised in industrial societies, we have generally been taught to ignore and hide our embodied processes rather than learn from them.[2] This differs greatly from many nonindustrial indigenous societies, in which people are encouraged to take time in ritual or meditation to delve inward and develop their body knowledge. In many contemporary traditional societies, self-reflection and aligning with inner guidance are considered important aspects of maturing and becoming an adult. Among the Oglala Sioux Indians, newly menstruating girls go through a traditional rite of passage in which they are mentored by a female mystic who helps them learn to connect with their inner knowledge and balance the powerful energy of menstruation to bring about healing for themselves and their tribe.

I have helped hundreds of women establish rich inner dialogues using mind-body processes such as meditation, journaling, visualization, and expressive movement, and I know you are capable of creating clear communication within yourself, too. At first, the very prospect of establishing a dialogue with your body may ignite flares of fear, doubt, and guilt. You may be afraid of what you may hear. You may doubt that you will be able to hear anything. Or you may feel guilty for having ignored your body's knowledge for so long. It is important to realize that the fear of facing your own inner truth will feel more uncomfortable and daunting before you go inward. Once you begin establishing an authentic relationship with your body using the exercises in the book, you will gradually experience more peace and confidence.

True integrative healing will assist you in learning to honor your total knowledge, not just that which flows from your mind. From this place of presence, you will tap into tremendous power and knowledge on how to care for and heal yourself. Simply embarking on this process will help awaken you to the vast wisdom that your body, mind, and spirit already contain. By opening up to the power of your knowing, rather than trying to crush your awareness through habitual processes of constriction and control, you free your vital energy and create pathways for profound healing on every level of your being.

The Gift of Energy

Another valuable contribution from integrative medicine is the acknowledgment of life energy in creating and maintaining health. Biomedicine has long ignored the existence of life energy or life force in relation to the body and healing. However, studies in other scientific fields during the last fifty years confirm the mind-body assertion that energy flows through all of life, affecting our bodies, our health, and even matter that appears to us as solid. While we wait for Western medical practices to fully incorporate these revelations from scientific disciplines such as physics, holistic practices provide a road map for how to tap into this invisible energy that is so essential to life and wellness.

Most complementary approaches recognize the importance of restoring and balancing energy as a key component of health. Receiving nourishing energy is particularly important for women's vitality. Many non-Western traditions state that feminine energy is about *receiving*. However, most of us in the West have been taught that feminine energy is about *giving*. As Western women, we are taught to give fully of ourselves without regularly taking the time to rest and rejuvenate. Our society has forgotten that to be able to give and give and give as most women do, you must first receive. Failure to do so leaves one depleted and exhausted. I believe that it is this cultural amnesia about the importance of receiving nourishing energy that has left so many of us ill, worn out, or in chronic pain for most of our adult lives. Our difficulties receiving energy may even influence our frequent inability to fully experience sexual pleasure or orgasm.

The good news is that we can change this. It is part of our journey as women to feel good about receiving energy, love, and pleasure without guilt, fear, or worry. We can learn from the many indigenous cultures that recognize the importance of women having emotional space to rejuvenate and rest as a necessary component of uterine wellness. Women in these cultures work very hard, yet they are aware of the importance of restoring and balancing their energy as a part of overall wellness rather than going and going until illness causes us to stop, which is a common occurrence in our society.

All the modes of holistic health I encourage you to explore provide ways to increase your ability to receive healing energy and become more balanced in your body. We allow in more nourishment when we support our bodies through healthy self-care practices, exercise, empowering beliefs, and relationships. This book is full of integrative practices such as conscious breathing, stress reduction, and whole-foods nutrition that will help you heal uterine imbalances and become more present in your body. If you begin to implement the mind-body practices now that help you tap into your inner knowledge and support your uterine health, you can prevent further problems with your uterus later in your life.

CHAPTER TWO

Your Uterus:
A Road Map

Mind-body modalities consider the uterus to be an integral component of women's total health. In contrast, the male-dominated field of medical research has rarely studied the uterus other than for its role in reproduction. However, the women's health movement has helped bring to light empowering new insights about the uterus and women's bodies. There are still relatively few investigations that explore nonreproductive uterine function, but the ones that do exist reveal that the uterus enhances multiple aspects of women's health. The uterus is important hormonally, protecting our heart health and keeping our blood from clotting. It plays an essential role in our anatomical structure and posture, providing support to help us move with ease. The uterus can also add to our sexual enjoyment and our ability to have pleasurable sensations in the vagina and cervix and the entire pelvic area.

This new understanding of the expanded nature of uterine function validates the holistic nature of our bodies. Everything is interconnected. If your uterus is depleted or removed, it cannot function properly to help create wellness in other areas of your body. It is vital to take care of your uterus as part of maintaining your overall health. This chapter provides a brief overview of the nonreproductive physiology of the uterus, highlighting the ways the uterus can help enrich your physical, sexual, and emotional health. It also outlines healthy lifestyle choices that support uterine wellness.

Scientific knowledge can take a long time to be integrated into standard medical practices. Many well-meaning physicians have been trained to consider the uterus as significant only for childbearing. We do not yet fully know the advantages that the uterus may provide for women's well-being, but recent discoveries are promising enough to inspire effective measures to reduce the high rates of uterine removal in the United States.

A Remarkable Organ

As we begin our journey to optimal uterine wellness, it is important to have a basic understanding of the uterus. The uterus sits in the center of the lower pelvis. It has two main sections: the upper, wider portion of the uterus is called the corpus or uterine body, and the lower, smaller portion of the uterus is the cervix. The top of the uterine body is named the fundus. At either side of the fundus the uterus attaches to the fallopian tubes. The fallopian tubes connect the uterus to the ovaries and serve as the pathway for the eggs to move from the ovaries to the uterus. The cervix is narrow, with a small opening that connects the uterus to the vagina. The bladder affixes to the uterus at its lower front segment.

The uterus has three distinct layers. The innermost lining of the uterus is called the endometrium. During the reproductive years of a woman's life, this mucous membrane layer either is shed during menstruation or becomes the nutrient-rich home in which an embryo implants for pregnancy. The middle layer of the uterus is called the myometrium, a thick layer of smooth muscular tissue that assists in the birthing process. The outside layer of the uterus, called the serosa, is a thin membrane that attaches to the uterine ligaments and pelvic connective tissue to hold the uterus in position in the pelvis.

The shape of the uterus is often described as an upside-down pear that becomes more rounded, like an apple, in women who have previously given birth. It is a muscular, hollow organ, typically three to four inches by two and a half inches—but this can vary due to age, presence of fibroids, or pregnancy. This normally small organ is capable of phenomenal feats. During pregnancy, the uterus dramatically expands to five times its original size, as its weight multiplies twentyfold to accommodate the fetus. It then miraculously and neatly shrinks back to its normal size within just six weeks after birth. The uterus is the only organ in the body that healthily undergoes such major transformation in size and shape.

Along with housing some of the strongest muscles in the body, the uterus has astonishing stamina. With an implanted embryo, the uterus can carry a healthy pregnancy to term even in a woman who is well past menopause. Women in their sixties have given birth to children. The oldest record of a woman giving birth in recent history is seventy.

Scientists view many of the amazing properties of the uterus as largely responsible for allowing humans to evolve as successfully as we have. During pregnancy, the uterus develops the placenta, which supplies a complete life support system for the fetus. The uterus and placenta perform all major functions essential for embryonic growth and development, such as providing nutrients and oxygen and clearing waste. The uterus nurtures and protects each fetus so exquisitely that we are able to develop the large brains that are the signature trait of our species.

The uterus endows us with many other important functions beyond our capacity for expansive intellect. The uterus is attached to important pelvic nerves and blood supply that provide sensation and sexual arousal in the uterus, clitoris, and vagina. During intercourse or other types of vaginal stimulation, the uterus elevates and enlarges with each phase of sexual response to generate satisfying feelings for women. In addition to clitoral orgasms, some women can also experience uterine orgasms as waves of intense pleasure. Deep thrusting causes the uterus to produce secretions that create contractions during orgasms. Women may also be able to achieve these same gratifying sensations in the uterus through imagery, deep rhythmic breathing, or massage.

Researchers describe uterine orgasms as "earth shattering" and profoundly emotional, often occurring when there is a strong intimate connection with a partner. Relatively few women may experience the mind-blowing bliss of pure uterine orgasms, but some experts believe that this number is artificially low because it is based on experiments conducted in laboratory settings where it may be difficult to achieve the emotional connection that seems to be a significant aspect of these particular orgasms. Studies show that at least 30 percent of all women have blended, or g-spot, orgasms, which are a combination of uterine and clitoral orgasms.[1] Even women who do not have orgasms can have increased enjoyment from rhythmic uterine contractions during sex.

Many ancient cultures celebrated the sexual gifts of the uterus and recognized it as one of the main pleasure centers for women. Today's renewed interest in ancient Tantric practices encourages women to get in touch with the energy of the uterus to expand ecstasy and awareness. For most of us, it may take a shift in the way we relate to the uterus to open up to the sexual rewards it can give us. In *Tantric Sex for Women*, Christa Schulte guides women to place a hand on their lower abdomen over the uterus and either tap lightly or make circles on their skin to open up the sexual energy in the uterus and help increase satisfaction during sex, either while alone or with a partner.[2] It may also help to imagine the uterus pulsating in a way that brings immense pleasure.

Uterine orgasms, like all orgasms, are a learned skill that you can cultivate if you allow yourself the freedom to explore what your body enjoys in a setting that feels safe for you in every way. This may not involve intercourse or a partner at first, but rather erotic images and fantasies that turn you on and pleasurable sensations such as caressing and stroking. Experiment with what it is like to deepen your breath and envision your powerful uterine surges during sex or masturbation. Do whatever feels right for you without worrying about what you look like, whether it is normal, or what others might think. Know that you are completely capable of creating the emotional intensity usually experienced during a uterine orgasm even if you are with yourself. Pleasure is personal, and you deserve to have a wonderful relationship with your uterus and body. It will nourish you emotionally and spiritually and bring more fun into your life.

As the main organ in our pelvic core, the uterus is also vital in maintaining healthy alignment and function for our pelvic anatomy. The uterus helps keep the bladder in position in the front of the pelvis and the bowel in place behind the uterus. In the absence of the uterus, the bowel, bladder, and other abdominal and pelvic organs may become displaced, causing pressure, pain, and reduced function. Without the structural support from the uterus, prolapsed bladder and pressure on the vagina are common, and bowel and urinary function are frequently compromised. Hysterectomies can damage nerves in the pelvic region, triggering pain and incontinence.

The uterus also enhances ovarian performance. Surgically removing the uterus can impede ovarian function, accelerating menopause and creating depression in some women. The blood supply to the ovaries is dependant in part on the uterus. Dr. Susan Love also proposes that there may be an important hormonal connection between the uterus and ovaries of which we are currently unaware. Love describes the pelvic region and the body in general as an environmental ecosystem. She suggests that by removing the uterus we disrupt the whole ecology of a woman's body in the same way that cutting down trees in a rain forest will have detrimental effects on other inhabitants of that region and the planet as a whole.[3] Just as we now know the ovaries continue to produce valuable hormones beyond menopause, Love proposes that the uterus may manufacture vital hormones that support the ovaries and other organs.

The actual position of the uterus in the body is also crucial for maintaining healthy posture. From an evolutionary perspective, the uterus must stay in a secure position, because it provides a protected haven for developing offspring. Consequently, the uterus is held safely in place by a network of ligaments—strong cords that generally hold bones in position rather than surround organs. These ligaments affix the uterus to the spine, hips, and pelvis and connect it to the ovaries, rectum, vagina, and bladder. The broad and cardinal ligaments attach the uterus to the pelvic walls. The uterosacral ligaments connect it to the lower back. The structural network that the uterus provides creates ease for movement, sitting, and standing. The presence of the uterus helps give structural integrity to the pelvic bones. Cutting the uterine ligaments weakens the support in the entire pelvic region. After hysterectomy, women often report that their hip bones broaden—which can create pelvic, back, leg, and even foot pain if posture becomes compromised.

The uterus may also carry out essential immune functions. The cervix protects women against bacterial infections. In her groundbreaking article "Menstruation as a Defense Against Pathogens Transported by Sperm," published in the September 1993 *Quarterly Review of Biology*, evolutionary biologist Margie Profit proposed that menstruation also provides the female body with a defense against infection caused by parasites or bacteria that enter during intercourse.[4] Profit turned the scientific world on its head by describing the uterus as an organ of smart design that guards women against the pathogens transported by sperm, rather than a passive organ with very few benefits to women beyond reproduction.

Profit explained that menstrual blood contains rich immune cells and does not clot like other blood specifically so that it can purify the body from microorganisms that might otherwise cause us harm. The uterus regularly sheds its lining from the body in case it is contaminated with pathogens. She explains that postmenopausal and pregnant women have thicker cervical mucous layers that protect against potential infection from sperm. Profit illustrates that the uterus is designed to bleed more when it discovers infection and shows that other healthy types of uterine bleeding—during ovulation and after birth, for example— also protect women's bodies from pathogens. Gynecologists opposed Profit's work, for the most part. However, much of the scientific community embraced her innovative research in menstruation and other areas of women's health as brilliant, and she was awarded an exclusive Mac-Arthur award for creative genius.

The uterus protects the body in other ways as well. It produces hormones that support the heart and relieve pain. Until recently, the uterus was portrayed as a passive receiver of hormones, not an active manufacturer in its own right. Scientific thought concluded that endocrine glands such as the pituitary, hypothalamus, pineal, thyroid, thymus, and adrenals, along with the ovaries were the main actors involved in creating hormonal balance throughout a woman's life. These ductless endocrine glands were considered the sites where women's hormones were created before being sent to the organs. Newer research shows that the uterus, along with other organs, plays a role in endocrine function. The uterus, kidney, liver, pancreas, and gallbladder all contain sets of cells that generate hormones critical to women's uterine health. By removing and processing materials from our blood, and transmitting the newly processed hormones for use in our bodies, this diffuse endocrine system affects virtually all of our cells, organs, and bodily functions.

As scientists increase their understanding of hormonal function in many major organs, research has revealed that the uterus produces chemicals that benefit our health well beyond reproduction. The uterus makes prostacyclin, a compound that prevents unhealthy blood clotting as well as heart disease.[5] Hysterectomy eliminates this protective advantage and increases women's risk of heart attack.

The uterus produces chemicals that protect women from heart disease and high blood pressure. The uterus also generates more than sixty kinds of prostaglandins and enzymes. Prostaglandins are hormones that function in many different ways. Some types of prostaglandins encourage the smooth muscles of the uterus to contract while simultaneously influencing the smooth, involuntary muscles in other areas of the body. These uterine prostaglandins are thought to help prevent blood vessels from becoming too rigid, potentially protecting you from heart disease and blood pressure problems.[6] Some types of prostaglandins provide immune benefits through their anti-inflammatory and inflammatory effects on the uterus and in other areas of the body.

The uterus also produces opiates such as endorphins and other helpful pain-reducing compounds. Like most of the chemicals generated by the uterus, this plethora of pain relievers is probably very helpful during uterine functions such as pregnancy and birth. But considering the large quantities of opiates the uterus pumps out, we can surmise that these feel-good substances may possibly offer additional positive gains in other aspects of health as well. One possible scenario is that these opiates, like some kinds of prostaglandins, improve women's immune response. Research conducted during the past twenty years demonstrates that natural endorphins may perform key immune system tasks.

These natural opioids actually affect the development and function of immune cells and may directly influence the immune system.[7]

Scientists recently discovered that the uterus produces vast amounts of anandamide, a naturally occurring, cannabis-like pleasure-producing chemical that is similar to marijuana and compounds found in dark chocolate. Its name derives from the Sanskrit word *ananda* ("bliss"). Researchers are just beginning to understand the many effects anandamide has on embryonic signaling and implantation.[8] The fact that the uterus manufactures much higher concentrations of anandamide than the brain begs for more research to see whether this chemical might also be involved in female sexual pleasure or boosting women's emotional states.

This limited body of research gives us a tiny peek into the potentially vast scope of uterine functions. It is essential that more health studies follow in order to increase our understanding of additional ways the uterus enhances our overall health. This new knowledge of the importance of uterine physiology to women's wellness should make us rethink our current tendency to remove the uterus with such frequency for benign conditions. Hysterectomies may still be the best option for some women with severe uterine problems; however, many experts surmise that the majority of hysterectomies are unnecessary and put women's lifelong health at risk.

These promising findings also call into question the long-term effects of synthetic hormones such as oral contraceptives and hormone replacement therapy on these nonreproductive uterine functions. More studies need to examine how artificial hormones affect the uterus's natural hormonal production and determine whether it is wise to use synthetic hormones for long periods of time. In the meantime, I encourage you to implement the effective strategies discussed throughout this book to strengthen your uterus. The next section presents a summary of the basic steps you can take to prevent hysterectomy and support your uterus so you can fully benefit from its many valuable attributes.

The Cornerstones of Uterine Health

Right now your body is undergoing many sophisticated processes to create hormonal balance and support your uterus. For this balance to occur and be maintained, the various parts of the body must be well enough to correctly receive information and instructions from the blood in the form of chemicals and to be able to carry out these instructions with the right timing. There are several important steps you can take to care for your body and enhance your body's abilities in biochemical communication. You can balance your hormones and protect your endocrine system and uterus by reducing stress, eating healthfully, getting plenty of sleep and exercise, and decreasing your exposure to toxins and synthetic hormones. You can also establish effective communication with health care providers to help you get the best health care available.

Stress Reduction

Your beliefs and thoughts directly affect your biochemistry, influencing your endocrine system, organs, immune system, nervous system, cells, and molecules. The uterus is of course affected by this holistic dance that takes place inside of you each second. Hundreds of scientific studies over the past two decades confirm this mind-body connection. By decreasing stress and improving your mental and emotional outlook, you can support your uterine health—easier said than done, of course, but crucial nonetheless.

The human body has evolved over thousands of years to triumph over life-threatening events. In the face of perceived danger, the endocrine system sends cortisol, adrenaline, and other hormones pulsating through your bloodstream. Blood pressure increases and the immune system becomes suppressed as the body prepares its "fight or flight" response.

Early humans mastered their environment by reacting quickly and effectively to danger. Today, many of us induce this adrenal response in situations that are stressful, but rarely perilous: to meet a deadline at work, for example. Over time, this pattern of evoking the stress response several times a day can cause hormonal imbalances, cellular damage, accelerated aging, and disease. This behavior is so prevalent in modern life that researchers from the Centers for Disease Control suggest that stress-related illness may be responsible for 75 to 90 percent of all doctor's visits in the United States.

There are many tools to help you create a less-stressful life even if you are currently facing health challenges. Developing your inner resources by establishing empowering beliefs and attitudes is one of the most useful stress-reduction tools. Building a network of social support also helps greatly decrease stress and improve health. Social science research shows that health and happiness are contagious. Having a social network of friends who are healthy and happy greatly enhances your ability to cultivate wellness and reduce stress. Meditation, prayer, faith, and any other practices that deepen spiritual connection are also very beneficial for many people. Regular exercise, healthy nutrition, and ample sleep will help you stay more positive about your ability to manage your life, as will focusing on activities that are nourishing rather than stressful.

> Stress levels are based on our perceptions about our ability to cope in particular situations. People have different views about how stressful a similar situation is, based on their confidence in their own coping skills. You can manage stress better and protect your uterine health by developing coping skills that help you feel assured about handling the pressure in your own life.

Whole-Foods Nutrition

The nutrients in the foods we eat, the beverages we drink, and the air we breathe provide our bodies with the materials needed to create healthy cells and repair imbalances. Many of your body's cells are replaced on a regular basis. For example, you renew the lining of your intestines every week. By providing your body with the nutrients you need to build strong healthy tissue, you can correct uterine imbalances that currently exist and develop overall health and vitality.

When we were younger, we learned that the nutrients in the foods we eat provide the minerals, vitamins, and essential fatty acids needed to build strong, healthy bodies and stay well. However, many of us did not grow up eating in ways that provide balanced nutrients to our bodies on a regular basis. As adults, women do not always hear from doctors about nutritional healing in relation to uterine wellness, even though professional guidelines encourage gynecologists to discuss nutrition as a preventative tool for menstrual and menopausal symptoms. Consequently, many women may not realize that nutrition can be an excellent tool to help heal and prevent uterine health problems.

Indeed, in my research observing hundreds of doctor-patient consultations on women's health, I rarely witnessed physicians discussing nutrition with their women patients. Unlike some medical fields, such as internal medicine or family practice, that use nutrition as one of the central methods for preventing and managing diseases such as diabetes, heart disease, and high blood pressure, many gynecologists generally focus on surgical or pharmaceutical approaches to uterine health problems. However, there is significant scientific research that clearly shows how proper nutrition can decrease uterine health problems. The human body has evolved to use whole foods to provide us with vitamins, minerals, and fats that are needed for many specific body processes with very few risks. When we do not give our bodies these crucial building blocks, we lack the materials needed to balance our hormones or support our uterine and immune function.

Diets filled with refined foods are low in nutrients and high in sugar, disrupting the endocrine system, increasing inflammation, and creating imbalances in the uterus. Continual lack of nutrient support significantly reduces pituitary, pineal, and hypothalamus function. These eating habits can eventually lead to a whole host of uterine problems, including PMS, infertility, endometriosis, and increased menopausal symptoms.

The chemicals commonly found in our contemporary food supply may also contribute to hormonal imbalances in women. High levels of chemicals from pesticides used to grow conventional fruits, vegetables, and grains negatively affect the uterus. The Environmental Protection Agency warns that people are exposed to large amounts of toxins from meat and dairy. Women who consume large quantities of meat and dairy raised with growth hormones and high levels of unhealthy fats often develop excessive estrogen conditions, such as endometriosis and uterine fibroids.

You can experiment and observe how you feel when you eat a wide variety of organic natural foods high in nutrients that your body can easily absorb instead of consuming mainly processed foods low in nutrients and high in sugars. In chapter four, I will provide an eating plan that naturally increases your nutrient intake, balances hormones, reduces inflammation, and supports uterine health. The nutrition sections in each subsequent chapter will build on these recommendations to support you in using nutrition to heal or prevent particular uterine issues.

Sound Sleep

Even a few nights of sleep disruptions or deficits can rewire the brain to produce fearful fight-or-flight responses that mimic psychiatric disease. Scientists believe that lack of sleep is strongly connected to serious health disorders such as diabetes, obesity, hormone imbalance, chronic illness, and suppressed immune function. These hormonal imbalances can weaken the endocrine system and compromise uterine health.

Most people in the United States get six or less hours of sleep each night, even though adults need eight to nine hours to be fully rested. Millions of people experience chronic sleep disorders, frustrating their attempts to get that elusive good night's sleep. On average, American women have more difficulties with sleep than men, adding to the uterine health crisis we are experiencing.

If you experience difficulties sleeping, give yourself permission to go to bed at a reasonable hour and get all the rest you need on a regular basis. An ideal bedtime is between 9 and 10:30 P.M. This gives your system a chance to recharge and lets your liver and adrenal glands recover and restore from a busy day. Your work and to-do list will wait until tomorrow, and you will be more aware and better able to focus if you are well rested. Sleep at least seven and a half hours, but preferably more, to help regulate blood sugar levels, prevent cravings, and have more energy.

Consider reducing or eliminating caffeine or consuming it only during the morning. Avoid alcohol, TV, computer work, email, stimulating books, and anything that gets you too charged up right before bedtime. Instead, engage in soothing activities that will help you unwind before bed, such as deep breathing and meditation. Sleep in a calm, dark, comfortable room. Employ the stress-reduction techniques in the Optimal Uterine Health Plan (part two) to help you get in touch with your feelings and balance your energy. Journal on how you can sleep better and explore what you can let go of on an emotional level to help you relax and feel worthy of truly nourishing yourself through a good night's sleep.

Nourishing Exercise

Healthy exercise is an important component in maintaining or restoring uterine health. Choose exercise that is fun for you and easy to fit in to your schedule. Walk with a friend, join a health club, or exercise in the privacy of your own home for thirty minutes or longer four times a week or at least for several minutes a day. Any kind of movement will help you feel better and have more energy. Add weight-bearing exercises to your workout routine to build muscle strength and prevent osteoporosis. If at any point you experience excessive fatigue or pain from exercise, listen to your body. See your doctor and scale back your intensity or find a different kind of movement that feels better.

Engaging in expressive forms of mind-body exercise such as yoga, dance, and tai chi can have surprising results in improving both mind

Frequent moderate exercise can decrease symptoms related to PMS, menopause, uterine fibroids, and endometriosis and can decrease stress—making it easier to take good care of yourself.

and body health. One of the most positive aspects of expressive mind-body exercise is that anyone can participate, regardless of physical activity level. Dance, tai chi, yoga, and other forms of expressive movement have shown significant psychological, mental, and physical benefits, even for people with physical limitations or severe health problems.

Chapter five outlines specific exercises that can help reduce a variety of uterine symptoms. It also discusses mind-body movement programs that help improve posture, decrease stress, and ease pelvic pain. Physical activity level is one of the main differences between non-Western and Western women. Being more active may play a big role in lowering rates of benign uterine disease. Women in non-Western societies don't go to the gym or consciously work at looking fit, but they typically move much more in their daily lives.

Detoxify

A growing body of evidence demonstrates that environmental toxins negatively affect our health. Of the thousands of chemicals that have been invented over the past sixty years, the compounds considered to have some of the most damaging effects on endocrine and uterine health are called endocrine disruptors. Endocrine disruptors are synthetic chemicals that mimic natural hormones when absorbed by the body.

Endocrine disruptors can interfere with hormonal levels, alter chemical pathways, encourage unbalanced hormone production, or block hormone production altogether. These compounds interfere with the body's sophisticated communication process and affect many important bodily functions, such as brain and reproductive development. Most of us living today have at least some levels of these undesirable toxins in our cells. Endocrine disruptors include DDT, PCB, dioxin, DES, bisphenol-A, phthalates, parabens, PBDE, some pesticides and herbicides, and some heavy metals. They are by-products of consumer products such as plastics, paper, dyes, and cleansers, as well as the chemicals used on our lawns, homes, and agriculture system. Many of these substances enter the body through our food, cosmetics, air, and water as well as contact with our clothes and furniture.

Surprisingly, most chemicals are not highly regulated when they enter the market. Efforts have begun to increase government supervision of endocrine disruptors, but for the time being you need to educate yourself and reduce your contact with these chemicals as much as possible. Eliminate pesticides in your home, yard, and garden. Use natural cleaning products. Purchase organic food as often as possible, or grow your own. Put filters on your kitchen faucet and showerhead to reduce your chlorine exposure.

Many plastics contain endocrine disruptors. Do not heat or store food in plastic containers—use glass instead, when possible. Some scientists warn against freezing food or water in plastic as well. Eliminate plastic water bottles that contain any endocrine disruptors. Make sure that children's toys, bottles, and pacifiers are made with safe chemicals.

Reduce your chemical exposure from body care and cosmetic products by using organic products. Chemicals in beauty care products enter the body through the skin, but the FDA does not regulate cosmetics in the same way it does food and drugs. The FDA states that except for color additives, cosmetic firms are responsible for substantiating the safety of their own products.

Many conventional cosmetics contain endocrine disruptors. Check the ingredients in your skin, hair, and nail products and discard any with synthetic chemicals, especially those with petroleum, phthalates, and parabens. Use only cosmetics containing organic and natural ingredients. Follow the nutritional and stress-reduction guidelines in the Optimal Uterine Health Plan to give your complexion the healthy glow you desire.

Consider taking an active role to encourage better chemical regulation and greater availability of healthier products. Express your concern to politicians, and do not underestimate your consumer power. Historically, tampons contained small amounts of dioxin, a group of related chemicals that were a by-product of the bleaching process. Consumer concern about the impact of these endocrine disruptors on women's health persuaded the EPA and manufacturers to establish different bleaching processes that produce dioxin-free tampons.

Chapter four presents nutritional strategies for promoting your ability to detoxify. In addition to eating an abundance of fresh fruits and vegetables, my guidelines for strengthening your liver and digestive tract will help you cleanse your body of unhealthy chemicals. Plenty of exercise and sleep will also enable you to reduce toxins and take better care of your uterine health. In this day and age, it may be impossible to completely eliminate toxic chemicals from your life, but every effort you make is a step toward better uterine health.

Limit Hormone Use

In 2005, the World Health Organization's cancer agency determined that hormone replacement therapy (HRT) and oral contraceptives containing estrogen and progestin are carcinogenic. Some physicians dispute this classification, but many others have concluded that the long-term risks of these products on women's health outweigh the benefits. Still, millions of women use hormonal contraception or HRT, some for decades. If you use HRT or hormonal contraceptives, perhaps you can take this opportunity to consider alternatives that provide similar benefits without such serious health consequences.

In the last few decades of the twentieth century, doctors prescribed HRT routinely, believing that the assumed heart, bone, and mental health benefits outweighed the increased risks of breast and uterine cancer—despite the absence of long-term studies. As early results of initial long-term studies came to light, these previous claims were proven to be less reliable than originally thought. The Women's Health Initiative was suddenly terminated when findings revealed that HRT proved detrimental to heart health, increasing women's risks of stroke and heart attack as well as dementia and breast cancer. As I discuss in more detail in chapter ten, a few recent analyses have shown that HRT may be safe to take for up to five years and is generally effective at reducing vasomotor symptoms such as hot flashes, night sweats, and vaginal dryness.

However, critical questions about the efficacy and risks of HRT remain. Many physicians specializing in menopause no longer promote using HRT for longer than five years. For some women, lifestyle changes and mind-body treatments—such as the increased exercise, stress reduction, herbal medicine, and improved nutrition that I describe in the Optimal Uterine Health Plan—can decrease menopausal symptoms as effectively as HRT without many of the dangerous side effects of hormone therapy.

Women who do not get complete relief from lifestyle changes may want to consider looking into bioidentical hormones with their physician and a qualified pharmacist. Bioidentical hormones come from plants and are then altered to structurally match the estrogen, progesterone, or androgen naturally found in women. Each prescription is designed individually to give women microdoses of estrogen, progesterone, testosterone, or other hormones needed to restore premenopausal levels. Many women report restored energy levels and reduced symptoms when taking these doses.

Bioidentical hormones have not been tested thoroughly and unknown risks may exist. However, bioidentical hormones usually come in very small doses, so many respected physicians consider them safer than conventional HRT. I encourage you to first try natural remedies such as acupuncture, herbs, nutrition, exercise, deep breathing, stress reduction, or homeopathy to see if you can get relief through methods with few side effects before trying any kind of hormonal therapy. If you do choose to take HRT or bioidentical hormones, talk to your doctor to determine the best timing so that you receive the optimal benefits.

Hormonal contraceptives are available orally, as a patch, in a vaginal ring, or in shot form. They are a very convenient and reliable method of pregnancy prevention that physicians tend to recommend because they think women are more likely to take a pill or use a patch more effectively than other types of contraceptive methods that have fewer side effects. This type of contraception has many advantages and gives women tremendous freedom. However, in controlling fertility, these synthetic birth control methods suppress our natural cycles and may cause imbalances or serious health threats.

Hormonal contraceptives—whether used for birth control, to eliminate acne, or to reduce menstrual or endometriosis pain—deplete our bodies of essential nutrients. This can happen through a variety of pathways, the most common pertaining to drug metabolism. Generally, the liver needs additional B vitamins, zinc, and vitamin C to process synthetic contraceptives. Years of using larger-than-normal amounts of these vitamins and minerals to metabolize contraceptives and the steroids they contain can result in deficiencies in the body.

Oral contraceptive use can impede muscle growth, even in women who exercise. Long-term contraceptive use also can foster yeast overgrowth that can create or exacerbate health problems such as chronic vaginal infections, digestive disorders, PMS, pelvic pain, and migraines. If these hormones compromise uterine and digestive health, it is reasonable to consider that they may also weaken endocrine and immune functions—potentially impairing other areas of your health.

In many cases, the synthetic hormones prescribed to women to improve conditions such as painful periods or acne can actually diminish overall wellness or create other health problems. You will vastly improve your health if you take a holistic, preventative approach to the uterus rather than relying only on treatments that do not correct the underlying chronic imbalances that caused the disease in the first place. Follow the suggestions I provide in the Optimal Uterine Health Plan and chapters six through eleven to help you learn how to effectively improve or prevent uterine conditions without putting your long-term health in jeopardy. To correct problems with your skin, follow the stress-reduction and nutritional recommendations in chapters three and four. Most people can reduce acne naturally by eliminating unhealthy fats and refined sugars and carbohydrates while restoring healthy bacteria to the intestines and getting plenty of beneficial fats as I describe in chapter four.

Consider using barrier contraceptive methods such as male and female condoms, diaphragm, natural family planning, cervical cap, sponge, or IUD if you have previously given birth. If you have a willing partner, let him be responsible for birth control at least some of the time. If you no longer wish to have children, he may want to consider having a vasectomy if he is comfortable with the potential health risks. The

Chinese have recently developed an effective birth control pill for men. If it becomes approved in other countries, this could be a good way for male partners to share birth control duties and reduce women's decades-long use of hormonal contraceptives. If you do not have a regular partner who is exclusively involved with you, use a barrier method for pregnancy prevention that simultaneously prevents sexually transmitted infections such as HIV.

If you do choose to use either HRT or hormonal contraceptives because of their many conveniences, follow the guidelines in the Optimal Uterine Health Program to provide your body with the support it needs to replenish the nutrients typically lost from long-term hormone use. You may want to use additional herbal liver supports such as milk thistle and dandelion and regularly follow whole-food nutritional detox-ification programs to strengthen your body's ability to metabolize medications. Always get regular Pap tests to detect any cervical irregu-larities and reduce your risks of developing cervical cancer. Don't beat yourself up or feel guilty about your choices. Instead, empower your-self by taking steps to stay healthy so you can fully enjoy the benefits of any medication you choose to take. Only you know what is best for your body. Employ the visualization techniques throughout this book to pic-ture any medications, your body, and all of your uterine functions work-ing in harmony.

Establish Effective Doctor-Patient Communication

Clearly communicating your questions, concerns, and goals to your physician is an equally important step in caring for your health. Take a current record of your health history, including allergies, procedure dates, test results, dates of recent menstrual cycles, and a symptom jour-nal documenting the frequency and severity of any problems you have been experiencing. Always include a list of current medications and any additional vitamins, supplements, or complementary treatments you may be undergoing.

Write down all of your questions and concerns before your appoint-ment and take your notes with you. Be clear on your goals for each appointment, and let your doctor know if you have specific concerns or objectives you would like to address. Write down useful information during your appointment. If you are considering an important procedure or treatment and would like someone to be there with you to help recall important details, take a friend or family member along.

Choose a physician with whom you feel comfortable talking honestly, whose communication style works well with your own. You will need to frankly reveal important personal information to your doctor. Gynecologists deal on a daily basis with the kind of issues you might be embarrassed about; it is a fundamental part of their job. The sooner you disclose any concerns or questions to your doctor, the easier it will be for him or her to help you resolve the problem. Your physician will also know about new treatments that he or she can use to help you heal any condition before it gets worse.

If you are not completely clear about what your doctor is telling you, ask her or him to clarify. Always ask what all the alternatives for a particular treatment or procedure are and for information about the research that supports and opposes your doctor's recommendations. Let your physician know that you want to fully understand all the different ways you can support your health. Request additional literature, with descriptions and explanations that you can take home with you, that explains all treatment options available—not just the one your doctor prefers. Find out whether your physician will respond to follow-up questions by email.

If the doctor does not have enough time to answer all of your questions, request a meeting with a patient educator or nurse. If you feel your questions are not sufficiently answered, your gynecologist doesn't spend

Ask your gynecologist to meet with you while you are fully dressed (either before or after your exam) so you feel more comfortable expressing yourself and asking questions than you might while undressed.

enough time with you, or you do not like or trust your doctor, find another one. If there are multiple doctors in the practice you go to and you prefer one or some over the others, request these doctors and make appointments far in advance, if needed and possible, to secure the physician you like. If you are concerned about missing work for frequent health care appointments, schedule yourself as your doctor's first appointment in the morning or immediately after lunch, if possible, to reduce your waiting time. Get recommendations from friends, support groups, or other women who have had good experiences with their doctors.

Establish Lifelong Wellness

Integrating these general health fundamentals into your life will enhance your uterine health. The Optimal Uterine Health Plan presented in the next three chapters provides you with many effective strategies and treatments. Choose techniques that resonate for you and will be easiest to incorporate into your life. Gradually add new practices into your routine each week, but do not attempt to change your life overnight. Be gentle with yourself and refrain from becoming judgmental about your progress. Do what feels right, and always celebrate your accomplishments.

It is my intention that this book will enable you to fully understand and support your uterine functions and discover new ways to heal any problems you may have. The uterus represents an important component of women's health that we can take care of and maintain in the same way we take care of our bones and hearts through beneficial lifelong practices. Use the Optimal Uterine Health Plan to prevent uterine imbalances and strengthen uterine processes so that you can create optimal wellness throughout your life.

PART TWO

The Optimal Uterine Health Plan

CHAPTER THREE

Transforming the Mind: Breathwork, Visualization, and Cognitive Restructuring

In Beijing, as I walked through the city each morning I was amazed to see parks filled with thousands of people silently moving in rhythmic synchronization practicing tai chi. I thought about how different this approach to greeting the new day was compared to the common Western routine of watching, reading, or listening to the news as we rush around preparing for work. I realized that the nature of our morning routines sets the pace for our days and symbolizes much about how we live our lives. Instead of balancing our energy and going deep inside to get in touch with our bodies, in the West we often begin and end our days focused on the external world and the problems in our lives. Stressed about work, family, and relationships, many of us rarely let go and experience true relaxation. Years of this kind of living take a toll on the body and soul.

This chapter will help you decrease stress and create uterine wellness through conscious breathing, visualization, and cognitive restructuring. Using effective tools to lower stress is vital to women's wellness, because chronic distress damages cellular tissue, disrupts hormonal balance, and fosters uterine disease. Research shows that performing daily relaxation practices reduces PMS,[1] painful periods,[2] and hot flashes[3] and can even increase fertility.[4] The relaxation techniques in this chapter enhance your physiology by strengthening your immune and endocrine systems while reducing pain and other symptoms that can occur during menstruation, pregnancy, and menopause.

The techniques in this chapter are a foundational part of my program because they will allow you to achieve the deep states of relaxation so essential for your body's healing and wellness. These practices will also enable you to understand and transform how your beliefs, thoughts, emotions, and stress levels influence your uterine health. You will integrate changes in nutrition, fitness, posture, and relationships more effectively if you first lower your stress and align your beliefs so you feel worthy of taking care of yourself. If you simply try to change your eating, exercise, and other self-care patterns without aligning your inner landscape to support you in your process, the suggestions I make throughout the book will not be as easy to implement. This is because beliefs create our reality. Whether you know it or not, your beliefs influence your thoughts and your thoughts shape the way you feel. In turn, your feelings affect your actions and your actions produce the results you get in your life.

If you transform your belief system to reflect that you are completely deserving of living a healthy, happy life, then you will be inspired to take the actions that create beneficial results for yourself. Reducing your stress will help you feel more empowered to take actions that nourish you. Deep breathing, meditation, and guided imagery can help soothe and revitalize the body, which will give you more energy for the changes you want to make. Visualization will also assist you in imagining the life you want so you can gain clarity about manifesting your goals.

Conscious Breathing

Conscious breathwork has been used in different cultures for thousands of years. Many mind-body healing traditions are used in combination with the breath. Breathing is one of the oldest and best-used tools for cultivating awareness, wellness, and connection to universal life force or energy.

At a fundamental level, breathing is about receiving energy. Women in the West have generally been socialized to receive nourishment with hesitation. We witness these patterns in our breath. Most of us take tiny little inhales and receive only enough air to keep us going, not nearly enough to fully oxygenate our cells, tissues, organs, and muscles.

If you notice this kind of restriction as you start to consciously breathe, ask yourself what it would be like to breathe in life more fully. Along with taking in fuller inhalations, you can begin the practice of receiving in many different areas of your life. Explore whether you can more easily receive a compliment. Observe whether you can completely receive a gift from a friend without worrying about obligations or becoming embarrassed. As you begin to inhale more deeply and easily, you will become more comfortable receiving love, energy, abundance, and nourishment in your life.

Just as we accept on every inhalation, we let go with every exhalation. Exhalations release stale air and free our outdated understandings or paradigms of who we really are. Each exhale liberates that which we no longer need, letting that energy pass back out into the universe to merge with its source. I encourage you to allow all of your inhalations and exhalations to flow naturally into one another without holding your breath, to help you develop the healthiest breathing patterns for lifelong health.

Breathwork for Uterine Health

In modern society, most people predominantly breathe into only a small area of their upper lungs and chest. However, to nourish the pelvic organs it is necessary to also breathe deeply into the middle and lower lungs to activate the diaphragm. When you practice this kind of deep diaphragmatic breathing you will be able to feel the air that you breathe inflating your abdomen. It is also possible to focus the deep breathing so that it expands your lower back and waist, but for most people it is easiest to start focusing deep breathing toward the belly first.

As an initial step to improve your uterine health, try to become more aware of integrating diaphragmatic breathing into your daily life.

Diaphragmatic breathing massages the abdominal muscles and tissues. It supports the pelvic muscles, connective tissue, and joints, and aids in the circulatory drainage of the pelvic organs. This results in improved digestive and endocrine function and greater oxygenation for the uterus. Deep breathing has been used extensively to decrease pain and ease childbirth. Research also shows that slow, deep abdominal breathing considerably reduces hot flashes in menopausal women[5] and when combined with meditation can improve PMS symptoms by 57 percent.[6]

It is important to continue to breathe into your chest (and upper back) some of the time. Breathing into every area of the lungs is essential for wellness and is one of the most effective stress-reduction tools available. Improved breathing not only strengthens the respiratory system but also relaxes muscles, supports immune function, improves mental capacity, balances the nervous system, and reduces pain. Follow the guidelines for diaphragmatic breathing in the next section daily to nourish your uterine cells, increase uterine function, and ease pain.

Diaphragmatic Breathing: To begin a deep breathing practice, choose an occasion when you will not be pressed for time so you can fully relax. Dress in loose-fitting clothing. Find a comfortable place to lie down, recline, or sit in a quiet area of your home. Conscious breathing may cause your body temperature to fluctuate, so consider having a blanket near you in case you cool down. If you tend to heat up while breathing, feel free to dress more lightly.

Begin by receiving some long, deep breaths to relax your mind and body. You can breathe in and out of your nose or your mouth—choose whichever is easiest for you. Breathing in and out of your mouth can be an effective way of quickly transforming your energy during conscious breathing exercises. However, breathing through your mouth all day long can cause imbalances, so normally breathe through your nose except while practicing conscious breathing. Breathe deeply and observe your breath.

Focus on your breath and notice how your body melts away any tension as you extend your inhalation to a duration that is comfortable for you. At the end of each inhalation watch your breathing flow naturally into your exhalation without holding your breath. Exhale deeply, letting go of all the air your body would like to release. Breathe deeply like this for several more breaths.

To commence diaphragmatic breathing, you will breathe into the lower and middle areas of your lungs. Place one hand on your belly and the other on your chest. Breathe deeply and see if you can breathe into the lower portions of your lungs to expand your belly like a balloon while your chest remains relatively stable. Notice how the hand on your abdomen lifts up as your stomach fills with air while the hand on your chest remains relatively still through this exercise. Take several inhales and exhales while you practice extending your breath more completely into your abdomen.

Experiment with lengthening your inhales and exhales as you become more relaxed in the breathing process. Learning to breathe into the lower areas of your lungs can take practice. Remind yourself that if you continue breathing consciously you will eventually breathe more easily. Even people with respiratory problems can achieve substantial benefits from learning how to breathe more deeply. You will also improve your uterine, digestive, and immune functions.

If you want to include your entire lungs in your deep breathing, you can combine diaphragmatic with chest breathing by slightly altering the preceding practice. Keep one hand on your abdomen and the other on your chest. On your next few inhalations, direct your breath into the bottom of your lungs, then to the middle section of your lungs, and finally to the top of your lungs. Use this same pattern during your exhales, emptying the air from the bottom of your lungs first, then the middle, and finally breathing out fully from the top part of your lungs. When you do this you will feel your abdomen and then your chest inflate during your inhale and contract while you exhale. Both of your hands will move as the air flows to the different areas of your lungs.

Uterine Breathing: For this exercise you can use whichever of the preceding diaphragmatic breathing practices is best for you. Just make

sure to engage your diaphragm and abdomen with your breath whenever you focus on your uterus. If it is comfortable for you, breathe in and
out of your mouth during this exercise. Breathing through the mouth is
an excellent tool for transforming the energy in your body, but I have
some clients who become light-headed during this process. If this happens to you, breathe in and out through your nose. Whichever method
you choose, make sure you receive full, long inhales and relax completely
as you let the exhale fall out of your body without holding onto it.

Breathe deeply into your abdomen and lungs and start directing
your breath into your uterus or, if you have had a hysterectomy, the area
where your uterus was. Focus on your uterine area for every inhalation
and exhalation. Imagine that the air you are breathing in is flowing
directly to your uterus or pelvic region. Feel that stale air or energy release
from your uterus or pelvis with every exhale, making more room for the
next inhalation. Let go of any judgments and enjoy the sense of peace
you may feel as you begin to fully oxygenate your uterus and pelvis,
increasing its function and circulation by breathing directly into it.

You may notice sensations of discomfort, tension, or fear coming up
in your awareness, your uterus, abdomen, or in the flow of your breath.
If so, give yourself permission to become conscious to your breathing
pattern for your next few breaths. Observe your breath and let yourself
know that breathing is not creating this discomfort; rather, it is only
bringing it into your attention so that you can heal it. If you begin to cry,
let the tears flow while you continue breathing. Crying is simply an
expression of energy, and deep breathing can help you release any energy
and emotions that have been bottled up inside you. Likewise, if you start
to yawn while you breathe, know that yawning is also an energy release,
so let yourself yawn as you receive full breaths and big exhalations.

Continue breathing deeply while you watch what is coming up in
you, returning to your breath and uterus or uterine area with every
inhale and exhale. Permit yourself to fully feel this emotion or energy.
Accept that this feeling is inside you, knowing that it will not overwhelm
you and that you have the power to let it go if you so choose. You do not
have to identify with this energy. Simply observe it while you stay with

your breath and keep focusing on your uterus or the area where your uterus was.

Breathing helps you become aware of the patterns inside you. You may prefer to continue this practice in the diaphragmatic breathing style described earlier. If so, know that simply being more present to your uterus will provide you with the insights and knowledge to heal yourself and create wellness throughout your life. Recognize that you may want to continue this breathing practice on a daily or weekly basis to support your uterine health.

If you would like to bring additional traditions to this breathwork practice, you can focus on transforming the energy you feel when you breathe into your uterus or pelvic region. Conscious breathing helps us access feelings and experiences we were previously so afraid to feel that we repressed them in our bodies. As you accept the feelings that come up for you during your breathwork process, reflect on the energies and beliefs you would like to bring into your body and life to replace that which is surfacing during your breathing.

The uterus holds our core beliefs about sexuality, creativity, relationships, and being a woman. If any of your beliefs or experiences about womanhood, femininity, feminine power, relationships, responsibility, creative freedom, and sexual pleasure have been too difficult to be present to, chances are you have buried them in your uterus or pelvis. This breathing practice is moving them to the surface to be examined by your conscious awareness. You can use transformational breathing to let go of nonnourishing beliefs and the feelings and energy they create in your being, and to open up to the truth about who you really are.

Continue breathing out these old frameworks that shaped your reality with pain, fear, and limits, while you inhale the beauty of your essential nature. With every breath, feel more fear and confusion empty out with the exhale while you breathe in love, health, and power with every inhale. Imagine beneficial energies flowing to your uterus and pelvis as you start to truly receive in each inhalation. Also, envision that any energy you want to let go of completely releases from your body, life, and home and goes out into the earth to transform into joy and light.

Breathe in and out of your uterine areas until you feel completely nourished. Most people will need to breathe for twenty to forty minutes the first time they do this exercise. Explore what your new beliefs feel like during your everyday life. What is it like to have a greater sense of freedom and safety in your uterus and pelvis? What feelings does being in your power as a woman evoke for you?

You may also want to use the Second Chakra Breathing exercise on page 129 and the Endocrine Restoration Breathing exercise on page 194. All of these breathwork techniques are usually practiced lying down in a peaceful setting. For some, breathwork can induce sleep, which can be beneficial in certain circumstances. However, if you tend to become drowsy or fall asleep during these breathing exercises, sit instead of reclining. You can also apply the concept of transformative breathing easily into your daily life. It can be used during meditation or even during activities in which you are physically active, like cleaning your house, exercising, doing yard work, or gardening.

Experiment with conscious breathing anytime you want to, throughout your day or evening. Research shows that just ten deep breaths several times a day can help you relax and improve your immune function. However, I recommend that everyone practice conscious breathing for ten minutes or more every day to let go of stress and fully relax. To decrease pain and accelerate uterine healing, use the conscious breathing exercises in this book for twenty minutes daily for at least three months.

> Combine your deep breathing with visualizations or intentions to breathe in qualities that you are welcoming into your life, such as wellness and vitality. Then use your exhale to let go of qualities you no longer want, such as powerlessness or disease.

Visualization

Visualization, also known as guided imagery, works by using sensory impressions to produce peaceful feelings. It can be performed in as little as five or ten minutes, yet it engages all the senses and creates powerful instructions and memories for the body.

Guided imagery is an important technique for uterine health because it is such an excellent way to initiate positive changes in your body's biochemistry. Your brain does not differentiate between visualized sensations and the experiences you have in reality, particularly when the envisioned images are focused on in a relaxed state. In both cases, whether stimuli are imagined or actually experienced, images cause your brain to send specific hormones to the different cells of the body. Thus effective imagery can lower your heart rate and blood pressure and reduce stress in just a few minutes. Through frequent focused visualization you can strengthen your nervous, endocrine, and immune systems, and create improved uterine health as well as emotional wellness.

Guided imagery relaxes your body and mind and connects you to your creativity, emotions, and inner wisdom. The deep state of awareness attained during visualization actually shifts your brain wave pattern out of the habitual, fast-paced beta rhythms and into the more calming alpha or theta levels. Alpha and theta waves are connected to right-brain utilization, the typically underused hemisphere of the brain that directs visual creativity and intuitive abilities. Alpha rhythms connect us to visual images; theta waves are associated with emotions, creativity, memories, and intuition. Guided imagery engages your right brain to tap into these important inner resources, enabling you to become aware of perspectives that you would not generally be able to access with standard left-brain thinking.

Guided imagery is particularly effective for reducing uterine pain. New neuroscience technologies have allowed researchers to understand why visualization helps alleviate many different kinds of chronic pain—even those that don't respond to standard medical treatments.

Acute pain is seen in the regions of the brain that are directly related to injured tissue. However, long-term pain shows up in the limbic system and prefrontal cortex, areas of the brain concerned with emotions and memories. Emotions and thoughts literally establish neural pathways in the brain. With chronic or cyclical pain, people's recurring emotions and thoughts about their discomfort strengthen these pathways, creating more pain in the body. In some cases, the pain can remain even if the tissue is healed, because pain impulses continue to move along these well-established nerve routes.

One gynecologist I interviewed suggested that much chronic uterine pain persists after surgery or pharmaceutical treatments because the nerve pathways are so "well worn" from years of distress. He explained that just like people who still experience "phantom limb" pain in an arm or leg even after it has been amputated, women still have pain impulses firing in their brains even after the damaged uterine tissue is repaired or removed.

Visualization and the other techniques in this chapter are excellent tools to stop this pain cycle because they help create new neural connections that bring pleasant rather than uncomfortable sensations to the body. Saturating yourself in good-feeling emotions through visualization will condition your nerve impulses to mainly travel along the new beneficial neural paths, eventually diminishing the chronic pain corridors in your brain.

Along with minimizing pain, visualization can have a powerful impact on the physiological aspects of uterine processes. One study used guided imagery to help college students lengthen the number of days between menstrual periods, in order to lessen problematic symptoms.[7]

Visualization is effective at producing a wide range of desired physiological changes, such as accelerating weight loss, decreasing cholesterol, reducing recovery time from surgery, and lessening anxiety.

Research in New Mexico demonstrated that during the postpartum period, women who used guided imagery for just four weeks scored higher on self-esteem measurements and significantly lowered their anxiety and depression.[8]

Visualization has also been shown to help people consciously balance their hormones. An investigation at the University of Miami determined that healthy adults can regulate hormone levels, improve mood, and reduce cortisol levels, depression, and fatigue by using visualization for three months.[9] My clients have successfully used guided imagery in combination with other strategies in this book to decrease hot flashes, alleviate fibroid pain, balance menstruation, and become pregnant. The chapters in part three present visualization scripts that can assist in improving menstruation, endometriosis, fibroids, fertility, and menopausal symptoms as well as surgical outcomes.

Even if you are not a highly visual person, you can use visualization. I have conducted thousands of guided imagery sessions with my clients. Some people connect most vividly to sights, others to sounds, taste, touch, scents, or simply through "knowing." It doesn't matter which sense you use to connect with your imagination, as long as it produces vibrant feelings for you. Allow yourself to be present with your process in a nonjudgmental way and discover what emerges. Focus on a feeling, sensation, image, or memory that creates positive feelings in your body and mind.

Visualization Rules of the Road

- Sense in the way that is the most natural for you.
- Allow yourself to truly feel whatever energy you want to expand in your life.
- Trust yourself and your ability to visualize.

The Law of Attraction

Visualization is based on the law of attraction. Quantum physics demonstrates that everything in the universe is energy. Even objects we normally experience as physical matter are made of pure energy at the most basic atomic levels. This includes you and me, this book you are reading, and the environment around you.

Everything is energy, and different energy has distinct vibratory frequencies that create the specific qualities we notice. The Law of Attraction suggests that the energy vibration or signature attracts more energy with a similar vibration or frequency. This is how molecules "fit together" on the atomic, subatomic, and particle level. Because we are all pure energy, the Law of Attraction applies to our experiences, feelings, thoughts, and bodies. Just like deep breathing, visualization is a tool that you can use anywhere. All it requires is your imagination and focused attention.

Visualization is one of the easiest and most effective ways to use the Law of Attraction to create what you would like in your life. When you feel, think, and believe a certain way, you create a particular energy vibration in your body. If your beliefs, feelings, and thoughts are dark, fearful, or anxious, you will attract more energy and experiences that match those particular vibrations. However, if you shift your energy through changing your beliefs and emotional landscape, you will shift the frequency you attract. It is virtually impossible to consistently "think positively" and attract beneficial energy if your core beliefs create significant fear, negativity, or self-deprecation. If you feel stuck, tired, or angry, be authentic about your feelings and use the cognitive restructuring and breathwork techniques in this book to reveal and transform the beliefs you hold that prevent you from enjoying life.

I developed the imagery exercises in this book to help clients and workshop participants create optimal uterine health. Each chapter in part three contains imagery that will help enhance or heal specific uterine conditions. The visualizations in this chapter are symbolic in nature and will be helpful for everyone. Symbolic visualizations can have profound healing effects on the emotional and physiological levels. They are also particularly helpful for establishing strong connections with subconscious levels of awareness. Give symbolic imagery a try—even if you tend to be very logical or cognitively focused. This will help you create more balance in your body by using both hemispheres of your brain.

Symbolic visualizations are very effective in illuminating negative beliefs about femininity and uterine health. Imagery helps you easily connect to your subconscious, where you hold many unacknowledged beliefs. It is these subconscious beliefs that influence many choices, decisions, and outcomes in your life. If you ever feel like you do not know why your life is not turning out the way you want it to, go to your subconscious and become aware of what is there through visualization, cognitive restructuring, or conscious breathing.

All of the guided imagery in the book will help you strengthen your uterine health. The visualizations in this chapter will help you open up communication with your body and enhance your energy—both of which are essential components for healing and creating wellness. See which imagery you are drawn to, then repeat each visualization numerous times. Allow your creativity to flow with all symbolic exercises. You may want to journal after doing visualizations, using the instructions outlined later in this chapter.

Visualizations can be as simple as imagining an uplifting image or symbol in your body or any area of your life.

- Envision crystal clear blue water flowing through you, clearing out nonnourishing energy or disease.
- Picture a beautiful symbol, such as a flower, at your uterus or pelvis.
- Imagine an empowering word such as "healed," "freedom," or "love" in your uterus, heart, or head.
- Visualize a word such as "tranquility" whenever you think of your home, office, or a particular person.

For each visualization exercise, select a peaceful setting where you can fully relax. Imagery is most effective when you do it in a deep meditative-like state, so refrain from practicing visualization when you drive or engage in any activities that require you to be fully alert. Wear loose clothing and either sit or lie in a comfortable position in a quiet area of your home where you will not be disturbed. Breathe deeply and relax your body by imagining that each breath is releasing tension, tightness, worry, anxiety, and fear from every part of your body.

Receiving Energy Visualization: This guided imagery exercise is very helpful for anyone who gets depleted easily. It is also great if you ever feel uncomfortable receiving support or habitually take on nonnourishing energy in your interactions with others. Begin by receiving a few long, deep breaths, imagining that you are breathing into every cell of your being. On the exhale, allow your breath to lengthen and your jaw to open wide, letting go of as much air as possible.

Visualize a golden sphere of light surrounding you. Set your intention that only nourishment can come inside this sphere of golden light, in which you are completely safe. Feel or know that the outside edge of your golden sphere is a beautiful golden filter that prevents nonnourishing energy from entering into your being or energy field. Envision that whenever nonnourishing energy nears you, it is immediately deflected by your golden sphere, and instead drops into the earth to be transformed into love and light.

With every inhale, imagine that you are breathing in nourishing golden energy. Know that this completely healing and benevolent energy is filling all of your cells. Hear or believe that every exhale is releasing all nonnourishing energy such as toxins, worries, stress, and disempowering beliefs out of your entire being. You might feel this as charcoal gray or heavy dark energy flowing out of you, away from your home, and into the earth. Envision that this nonnourishing energy transforms into love and light as it releases from your being. Allow yourself to receive all the love, energy, abundance, joy, and nourishment the universe has for you. Once you become familiar with this exercise, imagine rejuvenating golden energy flowing into your being any time you like. Visualize your golden sphere around you at work, in meetings, while on the phone, or during any interactions with people who leave you stressed or drained.

Uterine Labyrinth: Labyrinths have been used throughout history in many cultures to help people become better connected with their inner knowledge, truth, and purpose. Walking a labyrinth is a meditative process in which you can release the distractions of the outside world and contemplate the sacredness of your life's journey. I have used the labyrinth imagery with clients to help them get in touch with their inner knowledge.

A note about labyrinths: they are not mazes; rather, they are laid out simply, to help people go inward with intent. There is always a clear passageway in and out of a labyrinth, so you will never become lost.

Our bodies remember and store any past or present feelings that we repress and do not consciously process. This visualization can help you access memories held in your body. It may provide you with information about yourself to help you heal physical pain and emotional trauma.

You will create rich ways of accessing your inner guidance and power as a woman by using this visualization to create a sacred space in which you can safely explore the emotional memories held in your uterus. If you have had a hysterectomy, you can still do this exercise. Either imagine your uterus as it was before it was removed or focus your awareness on the space where your uterus was before surgery.

Lie down in a comfortable setting and breathe deeply in and out of your mouth. Feel your breath moving through you like waves in the ocean as you deepen your awareness into your body. Concentrate your intent on your uterus or in the area your uterus was.

Sense your uterus or uterine area inside you. Direct your breathing toward your uterus. Imagine that you are breathing into and out of your uterus for several breaths, calming your body and becoming totally peaceful. With every inhalation, envision that you are breathing in safety, clarity, and light to your uterus or uterine area. With every exhalation, envision letting go of confusion, doubt, or anger from your uterus.

Envision an entrance, opening, or doorway on the outer area of your uterus or within your pelvis where your uterus was. Before you enter, express gratitude for your uterus and acknowledge that you will honor it while you are there in this visualization. Visualize yourself entering into your uterus or pelvis. Notice anything you sense as you enter. You may feel a certain physical sensation or observe a specific energy or emotion. You might see a color, image, or person there or remember a certain memory. Ask whatever you notice there to tell you what message it has for you, knowing that you will remember it afterward.

Whether you experience anything in particular when you enter your uterus or not, allow yourself to go beyond this entrance into a passageway lit with the perfect amount of light for your comfort. Imagine that you are moving within a labyrinth, deeper and deeper, to the center of your uterus or your pelvic core. Feel yourself walking easily and slowly so that your pace helps you enter and maintain a meditative state. Breathe deeply and observe any sensations, images, sounds, or energy you experience during your visualization.

Visualize approaching the center of the labyrinth, which is aligned with the core of your uterus or uterine area. When you reach this most interior point of your labyrinth, envision yourself sitting down. From this point, open your awareness to any sights, sensations, sounds, smells, tastes, words, or messages. Remain open and ask your uterus or body whether it has any messages for you. Stay here as long as you want, breathing deeply and becoming present to the energy at the heart of your uterus or pelvis. Express gratitude to your body and uterus before imagining leaving through the labyrinth. Return your consciousness back to your body in the room and resume your normal breathing patterns.

Write down any insights you have from your experience. Repeat this imagery many times over the following weeks, even if no particular sensations came to you in this initial visualization. Some women in my workshops have described being able to access information about why they have fibroids, infertility issues, or other uterine problems. A few women have reported not having a deep experience initially, but with further attempts were able to get in touch with their uterine energy. Gift yourself with space and time to reflect on the information or experiences that emerge for you. The more you expand your awareness and delve into your subconscious, the more easily you can align your entire being and create the life you desire.

Future Imagery: Regularly envisioning joyous, healthy images of yourself will help establish beneficial neural pathways in your brain and disrupt habitual painful nerve impulses. Find a quiet place where you can lie down and become conscious of your breath. Breathe deeply on your inhale and exhale and connect with your body. Use your breath to become present and release all your cares and worries. Relax your body completely.

Picture yourself completely vibrant, nourished, and full of energy. See yourself as totally healthy in every way. Imagine the fun activities you will do when you are healthy and free of all pain. Envision your body and uterus fully balanced and in harmony. Visualize that your uterine processes actually enhance your health and help you be the wonderful woman that you already are.

Imagine how you will feel when you are completely healthy. Go ahead and sense the emotions that will be abundant in your life when you experience optimal health, such as joy, freedom, love, and gratitude. Allow yourself to fully enjoy these qualities inside your body now. Imagine sharing these qualities with those you love.

Connect to the renewed energy you are feeling in your body. Expand that energy to your heart, your head, your torso, your arms and legs, your feet and hands. Let yourself know that these new vibrations are healing you now and creating more vitality within you. Picture health, abundance, and success in every area of your life. Imagine growing older in perfect health and harmony. Stay with this imagery as long as you want, feeling the supportive sensations fully.

If you experience any hesitation or discomfort while doing this or any other visualization, use your breathing to help you release the fear that is coming up for you. Let yourself know that you can be healthy and that you do deserve wellness and happiness in every area of your life. If focusing on the future is not easy for you right now, use imagery to help expand the energies you want more of in your life today. Imagine that you can amplify and expand nourishing energies such as joy, peace, or vitality while you decrease the energies you don't want in your life. To do this, close your eyes and focus on one energy at a time.

Visualize that each energy has a particular color, feeling, sound, texture, vibration, or any kind of quality you can imagine. Begin by asking yourself, in the present moment, how big is the energy of fun (for example) in my life? Envision or feel how much fun is in your life. Is there so much fun that this energy is really easy to feel or sense (perhaps you might hear laughter)? Or if you could envisage the size of this energy in your life, would it be as big as you or as large as a house, or is there so little fun that the size of the energy is only a few inches wide? However you connect with the energy, go ahead and let yourself expand it by either picturing it getting bigger, feeling it becoming much stronger, or if you see it as a color, allowing the color to become brighter. Do whatever feels best to you to increase this energy.

Likewise, choose an energy you would like to release from your life, such as disease. Go ahead and sense, imagine, or picture how big or strong the energy of disease is in your life today. Allow yourself to believe that you can use guided imagery to reduce this energy and its impact on you. Visualize or feel that you can actually decrease the size, vibration, feeling, or power of disease by either imagining it shrinking, feeling it becoming weaker, or hearing it becoming quieter, while seeing yourself releasing the beliefs that have supported it. Do this practice daily until the unwanted energy and the beliefs that created its presence are no longer in your life. You can do this with any nonnourishing energies, always remembering to cultivate an energy you do want more of whenever you let go of a quality you do not desire. You may also want to use the Belief Transformation Visualization on page 213 and the Endocrine Gland Visualization on page 197.

Explore which visualizations help you feel most peaceful and revitalized. Feel free to use your imagination to expand or change the imagery that I provide or create your own visualizations. Like most practices, guided imagery needs to be repeated daily to be most effective. Use the guided imagery twice a day, for five to twenty minutes each time. Focus on the same sensory images daily for forty days or more. Even if you only have a minute or two each day to visualize, go ahead and visualize just for that minute, really connecting with the feelings that you want to expand in your life. A few minutes a day will help start to enhance your emotional state. However, to make physiological changes, most research recommends practicing guided imagery for twenty minutes twice a day for three months.

Cognitive Restructuring

Cultural anthropology shows that language and beliefs create the very fabric of reality for humans. Through beliefs, language, and thoughts we learn to view the world in certain ways. This socialization comes from our families and others in our immediate environments as well as the media, religion, education, and the culture at large. For most of us, our beliefs become the lens through which we view the world.

As we grow we are exposed to certain messages about ourselves, others, and the world. Socialization encourages us to embrace these shared understandings. Most of us will probably contest some of these beliefs, but we will accept others as truths—they become the way we think the world is. Many of these beliefs may be so deeply embedded in our subconscious minds that we do not even realize that we hold them. We assume they are facts, because everyone we know usually holds similar attitudes, or at least we think they do.

Consider a commonly held belief in American culture, such as "there is not enough time in the day." Although this statement may seem true to some of us, there are millions of people on the planet who actually regard time as abundant, cyclical, eternal, or unimportant. In my own anthropological research I have met people who do not think of time as scarce or even consider it as a major framework for organizing their days. I use this example not to assess which viewpoint is better or worse, but to begin to explore the power of our own cultural programming in our lives, bodies, and health.

Cognitive restructuring is the ability to change our belief and thought patterns to reduce stress and promote wellness. Research shows that cognitive restructuring helps decrease PMS,[10] and when used in combination with relaxation and education also reduces menopausal symptoms.[11] I have helped clients use cognitive restructuring to heal a wide variety of uterine issues. Establishing empowering beliefs will help you create health and manifest the results you want in every area of your life.

Conscious Creators

The way you think provides insight into your health patterns. Although it sounds simple, your attitudes and thoughts create your experience of the world. Your own views about your body, self-worth, and uterine processes may be affecting your health and ability to care for yourself more than you can imagine.

Do you take really good care of yourself when you are feeling well, or do you usually wait until you are sick to relax, get plenty of sleep, and make choices that truly support your health? Do you feel it is safe to make your own needs, wants, and desires high priorities in your relationships with others, or are you regularly putting others' wishes first? Can you envision yourself healthy and happy throughout your entire life, or do you think that your health will limit your quality of life now or in the future and naturally decline as you age?

Take a moment to reflect on each of these questions. Your answers will provide you with direct clues to your own inner landscape. If you generally wait to nourish yourself until you are sick or on the verge of illness, you are like millions of other women who delay fully supporting themselves until they are too run down to keep going. Why do we do this? Many of us hold deep-seated beliefs that a woman's job is to take care of everyone else in her life. Society has told us that we are nurturers. If this rings true to you, your opinions about your self-worth may be so tangled up with your abilities to nurture others that you often ignore your own self-care at the expense of your health.

Likewise, if you rarely place your own needs and wants before those of the others in your life, or experience considerable anxiety when you do, you may believe that love is scarce and conditional. Your attitudes will probably point to fears about what will happen in your relationships if you decide to express yourself honestly. Perhaps you think people will judge, criticize, like you less, or leave you. Or maybe at some unconscious level, you might suppose that there is power in being a martyr. As you consider your views you may find that you hold many different beliefs about the risks of showing up as your authentic self.

If you imagine your health necessarily becoming worse and limiting you as you grow and age, you may hold notions about your body that echo our societal attitudes of ageism. In societies where growing old is considered an honor, people often view elders as strong, healthy role models. In these cultures there are millions of healthy older people who still walk, work, and remain physically active daily. Even in our society, there are many examples of vibrant, healthy elders (you may be one of them), but we tend to think of them as the exception because they don't fit our stereotypical view of growing older in a society obsessed with youth. The idea that growing older automatically creates limited mobility and extreme health issues can create a self-fulfilling prophecy that shapes the way you age and grow.

If you share some of these common attitudes, the good news is that you can choose the beliefs you hold—even the ones that are buried deep within your unconscious. The tools in this book will help you become more aware of your mind-set so you can decide what you would like to maintain and what you would like to let go. Then you get to choose which new beliefs you will invite into your life to support and empower you.

Words, Thoughts, and Emotions as Guides

Beliefs have such power because they structure your way of thinking. Every day you think thousands of thoughts to yourself. You may contemplate gentle, compassionate, loving thoughts, or you may tend to berate yourself over and over again. Your thoughts and emotions are directly connected to the beliefs you hold. This is why it is so difficult to maintain positive thinking unless you establish nourishing beliefs first.

Your attitudes and thoughts produce powerful feelings in your body. If you believe you will never be healthy (or will never be loved, successful enough, or prosperous), you have many thoughts that support these attitudes every day. Every time you have these thoughts you will feel the emotions connected to the views you have. With these examples, you might feel angry, sad, powerless, or anxious. Whatever you are feeling, know that it is directly connected to your beliefs and thinking.

When you consider your emotions in this way, you can see that it is normal to feel depressed, angry, or sad when your thoughts and conclusions are pointing to a rather bleak reality or future. Instead of judging your emotions as bad or denying your feelings altogether, you can begin to examine the way you feel and explore the beliefs inside you that are creating these emotions. Honor all emotions as guides to your inner reality.

You can begin to untangle your identity from your thoughts and emotions by getting in touch with the beliefs that are causing them. Becoming present to your language and modes of expression can help you become aware of your beliefs. Notice how you talk about yourself, your body, your health, your life, other people, and the world. Pay attention to particular words you use. The way you speak will provide you with amazing insight into how you think, feel, and believe.

Do you frequently use "tired of" or "sick of" to describe how you feel about a certain person or situation? Words and thoughts have powerful energies. If you employ "tired" and "sick" in your language, you are attracting and amplifying those energies in your life. The next time you say these words, explore the beliefs behind your language. If your inquiry reveals a feeling of powerlessness, replace "sick of" or "tired of" with a statement about how you would like to change the situation or relationship. Try shifting the pattern of your words in order to establish more health and vitality in your life.

Examine how you speak and think about your health and your body. Do you tend to say harsh statements about the way you look, your uterine processes, or your fitness level to yourself or others? Does the way you talk about your health reveal a belief that you will find effective solutions and the right health providers to help you heal, or do your thoughts and statements stem from notions that you are going to have to suffer with your problems? See if becoming more attuned with the ways you can nurture yourself and seek assistance helps you feel better about your health. Instead of saying "fight this disease," release struggle as much as possible from your language and instead use statements that invite in wellness and healing, such as "I am taking the right steps to create health in my life" or "I am healing my uterus and my body."

Do you frequently use "should" in your language? Using the word *should* creates pressure and connotes judgment with the way things are. *Should*, along with *have to* and *need to* transform the energy of our choices into burdens and obligations. Explore how you feel if you release saying *should, have to*, and *need to* for a day or longer. You may find it helpful to use *get to* ("I get to go to the gym") or *choose to* ("I'm going to choose to eat better for the rest of the week") when discussing your goals, choices, and desires.

Listen to yourself without getting entangled in your emotions and thoughts. In this state of presence, you can begin to identify the beliefs that are creating your nonnourishing thought patterns and feelings. Then you get to decide whether you want to continue holding on to these old ideas or to create new empowering truths for yourself.

Cognitive Restructuring Tools

In addition to becoming more aware of your language, there are many other effective cognitive restructuring tools you can use to establish beneficial attitudes, thoughts, and emotions. Journaling is an effective way to unearth obscured beliefs. Stream-of-consciousness journaling has become popular in recent years because it lets your deepest beliefs emerge without criticism in a format you can return to again and again.

Begin your journaling process by letting go of all judgment about your writing. Breathe deeply for several breaths and focus your awareness on your situation, concern, or question and give yourself permission to write freely.

When you are ready to write, date your journal entry or image every time. Then allow the words to pour out of you onto the pages of your journal without even thinking about what you are saying. As you write, unleash a free flow of information without judgment or reflection. You can journal for a few minutes or as long as an hour—do whatever feels best to you.

To journal about your uterine health, begin by expressing gratitude for your uterus and for your body, even if you are currently experiencing uterine problems or have had a hysterectomy. Breathe as you start to connect to your uterus or uterine area. Imagine where it is in your body, what it looks like, and how it feels. Journal about what your uterus means to you. You may want to write about your inner beliefs and feelings about your uterine processes or any messages you have taken in from society, your family, or others about being female.

Write about any possible steps you can take to improve your uterine health. These might include how you feel about any treatment options you are considering or how you can heal any grief, anger, and sadness you may hold regarding your uterine functions. You can also journal on how you can improve your nutrition or create empowering beliefs, healthier relationships, enhanced personal power, emotional balance, increased sexual pleasure, and creativity.

You can also write a question or word such as *uterus, menstruation, menopause, pregnancy, hysterectomy, self-care,* or *exercise* in the center of a page of your journal. Underline or circle your subject and surround it with any ideas, phrases, or words that enter your mind. Additionally, you can draw pictures or make collages about your uterine health or any other subject you would like to explore, letting the images that come to you help reveal your unconscious views about a particular issue.

When you are done, before returning to examine your image or passage, take time to stretch, walk, and observe how you feel. Look at what you have written or created with an open heart. By having the courage to reveal, examine, and honor your inner wisdom, you become a conscious creator of your own reality.

If you have a serious uterine condition, journal on a regular basis. However, these exercises are beneficial for all women, even those who are quite healthy and are using this book mainly for its preventative awareness. Just as these methods facilitate healing of uterine imbalances, they can be easily employed for other sorts of health issues.

In addition to journaling, you may want to use the Four Steps to Change[12] process to establish supportive beliefs. This four-step process is one of the most effective cognitive restructuring tools I have found.

The first step of the change process is to recognize how you truly feel. This step entails being completely honest with yourself about how you feel about a situation you would like to change. If you feel sad or depressed, go ahead and delve inside to see if you are also angry or furious about the situation. Be completely real about how hurt, angry, and upset you are at yourself, your family, friends, work, the world, or even God. You do not need to tell others how you feel as you do this process, but it is completely essential that you allow yourself the safe emotional space to completely express all the hurt, anger, betrayal, and sadness inside you. Telling the truth to yourself will free up your energy to change your situation.

The second step has two parts. The first part is to acknowledge who created the situation. Since you create your own experience of reality, the answer to this will always be you. Even if someone else did something to you, you create how you *feel* about the interaction. Even in very difficult personal or societal situations, you always have the power to choose what you believe about yourself and how you feel. This is good news because it means you have the power to change what you do not like in your life and create a wonderful reality for yourself. This is not meant to initiate self-blame; rather, it's meant to expand your consciousness that you can always choose to believe, feel, and affirm your inherent infinite self-worth, value, and personal power.

The second part of step two is to acknowledge the beliefs you hold that led you to create your response to the situation. For most people there will be many beliefs. Some may be general or about other people, such as "the world is a difficult place," "people are mean," or "(someone) doesn't truly care about me." Beliefs about other people and the world are important, but it is necessary to get in touch with the beliefs about yourself as well. Personal beliefs might be "I'm afraid to let (someone) get close because I think they might abandon me" or "If I have too much success other people will be jealous."

All of these types of beliefs are illuminating and need to be recognized and changed in order to live a healthy life; however, the most crucial beliefs to get in touch with are "I am" beliefs, because they have such a huge impact on your identity. These beliefs are commonly "I am not safe," "I am not enough," "I am not worthy," "I am guilty," "I am bad," or something similar. Each time you do this exercise, try to come up with at least ten beliefs, two of which are "I am" beliefs. Journal or breathe on how these beliefs make you feel. Allow yourself to feel all of the pain that your beliefs have caused, so you can truly let it go.

Step three is forgiving yourself and anyone else involved in the situation. When you look at the beliefs you hold about the situation you want to change, you will see that your feelings and actions were appropriate based on what you believed. If someone believes that she did not deserve success or love or that she was not enough, it makes sense that she might not stand up for herself. You can go ahead and forgive yourself completely, knowing that you are now going to create empowered beliefs that will allow you to change your life. Feel forgiveness and love for yourself and others throughout your body.

Step four is to create change by establishing new beliefs and taking new actions to support your new beliefs. You are worthy of love, health, vitality, abundance, and joy—we all are, even though many of us don't recognize this about ourselves. Go ahead and adopt this and other empowering beliefs, such as "I am enough," "I am innocent," "I am free," and "I am safe." Breathe these new beliefs into your body. Identify any actions you took in the past that reinforced your old disempowering beliefs. For example, if you believed you were not safe, you may have withdrawn in public settings, become easily defensive, or consistently focused on other people to draw attention away from yourself. Begin to take actions that are the opposite of what you have habitually done. Taking new actions will help you see that you are safe, worthy, or enough, just the way you are.

Just as it is important to examine and change any unhealthy beliefs, it is equally essential to celebrate who you are and the success you already have. Honoring our successes daily is a great cognitive restructuring tool; it reverses our inclination to focus only on what is wrong in our lives or on our inability to make the changes we want. The Law of Attraction tells us that what we concentrate on expands. Take time to acknowledge or write down all the successes you have each day. Recognize any success—such as being kind to yourself, finishing a project at work, going to an exercise class, having a great night out with a friend, taking the time to breathe deeply, or simply being present.

We often treat ourselves harshly for minor mistakes, yet many of us tend to not take the time to appreciate our victories. Let yourself completely feel and enjoy your successes, whether they are related to health, relationships, work, spirituality, relaxation, or fun. Keep a success journal (or record your successes in your main journal) so you have an ongoing record you can look at to remind yourself of the wonderful energy you have created in your life. If you use this process when you try the suggestions in this book, you will find that you will have more fun and ease incorporating the strategies.

Unconscious Contracts

In *The Four Agreements*, Don Miguel Ruiz says that the words we speak represent unconscious agreements we have made with ourselves.[13] Observing your language, thoughts, and the way you treat yourself will help you become more aware of the contracts or agreements you have established with yourself and others. Many of us tend to have contracts that reinforce our loyalty to the views of our families and societies, often at great expense to our own health and happiness.

Perhaps you believe that uterine or breast disease is your destiny as a woman. Most Western women have been exposed to these beliefs through family, friends, the media, or biomedical philosophy. Many of us have either consciously or unconsciously agreed to accept the belief that the uterus creates suffering. Other women have agreed that their breasts will cause them harm. Even if you are not entirely aware of it, you may have learned and thus agreed that women's bodies are naturally problematic.

However, the fact that women in certain areas of the world have fewer problems with menstruation and menopause and lower breast cancer rates shows that uterine problems and breast disease do not have to be our destiny as women. These divergent epidemiological patterns suggest that lifestyle, nutrition, and the environment have an important impact on women's health. Biology is not destiny. Even if you have a family history of uterine problems, you can use the holistic health strategies in this book to improve your uterine health beyond what you may have previously thought feasible.

An important component of uterine wellness is lowering stress through conscious breathing, visualization, and establishing loving beliefs. It is important to develop agreements that optimal uterine health is normal and possible for you to have. The more fully you believe that vitality is your birthright, the more easily you will be able to incorporate the Optimal Uterine Health Plan into your daily life.

As you integrate these strategies, I encourage you to acknowledge your accomplishments and begin to make your own body your new best friend. Recognize yourself for all the ways you take care of yourself. Celebrate your successes, big and small, and imagine your power expanding in every part of your life. I know, from my own journey as well as my work with clients, that you will feel the energy of these changes manifest in your life in many wonderful ways.

CHAPTER FOUR

The Power of Food: Uterine Wellness Through Nutrition

Until quite recently in human existence, food served as a staple of healing. Traditionally, women passed down knowledge on how to use herbs, vegetables, fruits, whole grains, oils, nuts, and seeds to cultivate vitality and heal imbalances. During the past fifty years our understanding of food has shifted greatly as modern interests in eating became focused on speed and convenience. Much of the knowledge regarding the healing powers of food has been lost in Western society as we have come to rely on others to prepare our meals—which have increasingly declined in nutritional quality.

Women around the globe have known what to eat to balance their periods, decrease inflammation and pain, prevent menopausal symptoms, and nurture pregnancy. Whole foods can promote hormonal balance, release inflammation, and strengthen the immune system to reduce uterine symptoms and restore us to health. This chapter aims to help you reclaim some of that knowledge and inspire you to further your own awareness of food as a traditional resource for health and wellness.

Foods to Strengthen the Uterus

These dietary guidelines will help you create and maintain uterine health. You can nurture yourself with delicious, high-energy natural foods rather than depriving yourself of nourishment when you are hungry or filling yourself with empty or unhealthy calories. This book does not contain a weight-loss program. However, combining these healthy eating practices with regular exercise can help you release unwanted weight.

Your body is designed primarily to eat green leafy vegetables, herbs, fruit, nuts, legumes, fish, small amounts of meat, and no refined or artificial foods or sugars. Anthropologists now know that most early humans were not hunter-gatherers; rather, our ancestors spent hundreds of thousands of years mostly foraging and gathering plant foods that grew in their environment. Our bodies have not had time to adjust to the high intake of refined foods, sugar, salt, and newly developed chemicals introduced during the last century. Use the following guidelines to support your biochemistry and boost your uterine health.

It is fundamental to start to know your body in order to become familiar with which foods nourish you and help you feel better. Notice the foods that give you energy and the ones that create pain and fatigue. Keep a food journal to track how you feel after eating. You may feel the effects of some foods immediately after they have been digested, or not until a day or two later. If you think you may not tolerate a certain kind of food, eliminate it totally from your diet for at least six to eight weeks to test whether you feel better.

Eat an Abundance of Organic Vegetables and Fruit

The amount of estrogen in a woman's body is constantly changing and is directly affected by the foods she eats. Researchers surmise that the low amount of healthy vegetables, combined with the high amount of unhealthy fats, animal protein, and environmental estrogen in the standard Western diet, all elevate estrogen levels in the blood, contributing to our increased incidence of uterine disorders.

Vegetables and fruits are a better source of vitamins, minerals, and nutrients than supplements and some types of animal-based foods. Fruits and vegetables are also rich in antioxidants and phytochemicals that support healthy cellular structure and nourish the uterus. Numerous studies illustrate that diets with modest amounts of high-quality fats and plenty of complex carbohydrates, vitamins, and minerals from vegetables, fruits, and legumes decrease uterine pain and imbalances. Findings published in *Obstetrics & Gynecology* in 2000 emphasize that a low-fat, high-fiber vegetarian diet reduced PMS and pain for research participants.[1] A 2004 study of one thousand women in northern Italy found that women who consumed more green vegetables and fruit had a 40 percent lower incidence of endometriosis.[2] Vegetables and supplements rich in phytoestrogens alleviate menopausal symptoms such as hot flashes and night sweats.[3] Scientists are just beginning to study how nutrition can ease fibroid tumor growth and discomfort and the early results look promising.

Fibroid tumors, like endometriosis, decrease in size and symptoms as blood estrogen concentrations decline; eating more vegetables aids this process. Additionally, women with fibroids have an increased risk of uterine cancer and frequent digestive difficulties. The American Cancer Institute and other health organizations promote eating mostly plant-based foods as one of the healthiest steps people can take to diminish their cancer risks.

I learned about the healing effects of a plant-based diet firsthand by living in West Africa as a college student. Despite my family's best efforts, growing up I ate mostly meat, refined food, and sweets. When I moved to Togo, there were very few opportunities for me to eat anything besides

Dietary fiber from plants helps your liver cleanse excess estrogen from your blood. Adequate vegetable and fruit fiber literally sweeps out waste estrogen from your body so it is not sent back into your bloodstream. This fiber is essential for uterine wellness.

local organically grown vegetables and fruit and freshly caught fish. There was virtually no beef, chicken, or pork, and very few dairy products. Within a month I noticed that the chronic pelvic pain, bloating, and digestive problems I had experienced for years had disappeared, and my PMS symptoms were appreciably better.

On my arrival back to the United States, the first meal I ate consisted of some of my favorite foods—red meat, green beans cooked with bacon, mashed potatoes, bread, and pie with ice cream. To my dismay, the next day my abdominal pain was back in full force. There was no mistaking what had caused it—the very foods I loved. I didn't want to go back to the fatigue and pain I had felt for so many years. I immediately switched to a plant-based diet and gained a great appreciation for the power of food on my immediate physical health.

To promote uterine wellness, eat a rainbow of organic vegetables and fruits and avoid endocrine disruptors such as fungicides and pesticides. Organically grown vegetables and fruit are grown in richer soil often for longer periods of time than conventionally grown produce. Consequently, organics contain more vitamins, minerals, nutrients, phy-

Aim for nine servings of vegetables and fruit every day. The options below will provide ample antioxidants, phytochemicals, minerals, and vitamins.

- Eat plenty of leafy green vegetables like kale, bok choy, spinach, collard greens, chard, and beet greens, which generally have many more nutritional benefits than most lettuce.
- Try winter squashes such as acorn, butternut, and delicata.
- Eat broccoli, sweet potatoes, cucumbers, avocadoes, sweet peppers, tomatoes, and beets.
- Experiment with sea vegetables such as wakame and hijiki, which are easily prepared by simply soaking in water for a few minutes and are rich in minerals and nutrients.
- Enjoy papaya, pineapple, berries, bananas, plums, apricots, apples, and other fruits, either raw or stewed.

tochemicals, and antioxidants—even though they may be smaller or less attractive (by supermarket standards) than conventionally grown produce. Whenever possible, eat local produce. The fresher vegetables and fruit are, the more nutrients they contain.

When you do cook vegetables, roast, steam, or sauté them. Frying and cooking at high heat for long periods of time can deplete many of their benefits. Flavor vegetables with plenty of nutrient-rich herbs and spices—such as oregano, dill, rosemary, parsley, cilantro, garlic, and turmeric—in place of salt, margarine, or sugar. Use fresh herbs when possible, and grow your own if you enjoy it, so you always have plenty on hand.

> By paying attention to how your body feels, you can achieve the right balance of cooked and raw vegetables and fruits for you. Eat more raw foods during hot weather or if you experience constipation. Eat mostly cooked and stewed vegetables and fruit during cold weather or if your bowel movements tend to be loose.

Balance Your Blood Glucose Levels

One of the most important steps you can take to improve your health and prevent future uterine problems is to eat in ways that maintain relatively even blood glucose (sugar) levels. One way to help do this is to eat a good breakfast—daily. A 2003 study of female Japanese college students confirmed that women who do not regularly eat breakfast tend to develop severe uterine pain during their periods as well as digestive difficulties.[4] Women in the study who ate breakfast every day were generally pain-free and experienced healthy digestive and elimination patterns.

Eating breakfast may have produced such good health for the participants because, for one thing, the traditional Japanese breakfast foods help balance hormones. Many of the women in societies with low rates of benign uterine problems typically eat vegetables, whole grains, or small amounts of protein for breakfast. The traditional Japanese breakfast is miso soup with seaweed, vegetables, and brown rice accompanied by grilled salmon. This type of breakfast balances blood sugar and prevents PMS and other uterine imbalances.

In the West, many women either skip breakfast altogether or eat high-glycemic foods such as refined cereal, toast, or pastries, all of which increase blood sugar levels when ingested. All carbohydrate foods do not have the same impact on the body. High-glycemic foods create large fluctuations in blood glucose and insulin levels. Your body functions best when blood sugar levels are fairly constant. Consuming refined foods first thing in the morning or not eating breakfast at all creates unhealthy blood sugar levels throughout the day. When you skip meals or do not eat frequently enough, your blood sugar decreases. Low blood sugar results in fatigue, hormonal fluctuations, insatiable hunger, or cravings for foods that will quickly raise your blood glucose.

Increasing low-glycemic whole foods that contain complex carbohydrates and healthy fats while decreasing sugary and refined foods and beverages can reduce swelling, bloating, and breast tenderness for pregnant and premenstrual women. An investigation of women with endometriosis revealed that symptoms are in part a result of insulin and hormonal imbalances caused by eating too many high-glycemic carbohydrates and not enough healthy fats.[5] Study participants experienced a decrease in symptoms within two months of increasing complex carbohydrates and healthy fats while decreasing caffeine, high-glycemic foods, and the protein tyramine, which occurs in elevated amounts in aged, fermented, or spoiled foods such as hard sausages, smoked meat, and aged cheese and can induce pain in some people.

When I begin working with clients who have uterine health concerns, one of the first actions I suggest is to make breakfast a priority. Molly was a twenty-three-year-old hairdresser who experienced premenstrual headaches and feelings of anxiety for a week before her periods. Molly would generally have coffee and a muffin in the mornings or skip breakfast altogether. She was reluctant to eat a big breakfast because she was afraid the extra calories would make her gain weight. After I explained that eating in the morning generally helps women lose weight, Molly decided to eat a whole-foods breakfast for a month to see if it could positively affect her health. I encouraged her to get up earlier so she could eat an early breakfast and exercise before work. Within just a few weeks, Molly noticed an increase in her energy levels and less intense symptoms preceding her period. She continued to make healthy nutrition and lifestyle choices and actually lost weight with her new eating and exercise program. Molly took special care to eat especially well every two weeks before her period, which reduced her PMS tension and anxiety even more.

To help heal and prevent uterine problems and promote overall health, eat complex carbohydrates and healthy protein and fats for breakfast and lunch. Eating vegetables, protein, and whole grains such as brown rice or oats is a great way to start your day. Make enough veggies, fish, tofu, beans, or chicken for dinner so you have leftovers to eat for breakfast the next day.

If you frequently experience gastrointestinal problems such as diarrhea or bloating, you might want to explore eliminating gluten from your diet for four to six weeks to see if your symptoms diminish. Gluten is a complex protein that many people have difficulty digesting. It is found in wheat, barley, and rye as well as any food products made from these grains. Many researchers recommend eliminating oats from your diet as well because some oats may contain gluten through contamination. If you find that you are gluten intolerant, eat gluten-free whole grains such as quinoa, millet, pure buckwheat, brown rice, or certified gluten-free oats.

For a healthy breakfast, eat quinoa or oatmeal with sliced almonds sweetened with fruit and flavored with vanilla extract and cinnamon. Put sunflower seed butter with all-fruit spread on wild rice cakes or whole-grain or wheat-free toast. Have a couple of apples with some walnuts or hummus. Make smoothies with fruits and vegetables and ground flaxseed. Occasionally have free-range eggs poached or in a vegetable omelet. If you tolerate dairy well, try some plain organic yogurt with fresh fruit.

For lunch, eat a large portion of veggies accompanied with protein such as quinoa, beans, fish, grilled chicken, roasted turkey, or tempeh. If a portable sandwich is easiest, choose whole-grain or wheat-free breads and fill them with plenty of vegetables along with your protein of choice. In lieu of white rice, make satisfying whole-grain salads with herbs, protein, vegetables, and healthy oils and vinegars combined with short-grain brown rice, wild rice, millet, and buckwheat or, if you are not gluten sensitive, bulgur, barley, and wheat berries.

As you add in healthy whole foods for breakfast, lunch, and dinner, start to reduce refined and sweet foods and beverages. Explore eating a nonsweet breakfast at least once a week, then see if you can expand that practice to another day to retrain your tastes and expectations about which foods are best to eat in the morning. Consume the least amount of meat at dinner and aim to eat all animal protein before 7 P.M. every day to give your body plenty of time to digest before bedtime.

Reducing sweets, refined foods, and caffeine can significantly improve PMS, infertility, endometriosis, and menopausal symptoms. Sodas and other sweet drinks are the largest source of calories for Americans. In addition to wreaking havoc on blood glucose levels, processed sugar causes the overgrowth of unhealthy yeast and fungi in the intestinal tract, compromising digestive health. The phosphorus in soft drinks (even those sweetened with artificial sweeteners) leaches calcium from the body, with negative effects on menstrual and bone health. Cutting down on—or eventually eliminating—sodas, caffeine, and other sweet drinks and food can significantly help to heal or prevent uterine issues.

Refined foods have been stripped of most nutrients, vitamins, and minerals that nourish your uterus. Manufacturers often enrich refined wheat and white flour products because they are so depleted of nutrients, but these added nutrients are synthetic and not as easy to assimi-

- Partake of healthy mini meals in the midmorning and afternoon if you are hungry.
- Do not wait until you are starving to eat lunch.
- Eat dinner early; if possible, between 5 and 7 P.M.

late as the vitamins and enzymes found in whole foods. Processed foods generally have high sodium levels that can cause premenstrual or pregnancy swelling and breast tenderness. Wheat products may also disturb magnesium and zinc levels, which can cause uterine pain. Researchers in England found that 80 percent of women with endometriosis could ease or eliminate their pain by removing wheat from their diet.[6]

At times when you would regularly have something sweet, refined, or caffeinated to energize you, stretch, walk around, or do some deep breathing for a few minutes. Eat a whole-foods snack, such as an apple and some walnuts, that will invigorate you without the subsequent crash you get from processed foods and drinks. Get more sleep and use stress-reduction techniques such as the visualization and breathing exercises in this book to have more energy without depending as frequently on caffeine.

As you begin to replace refined foods, think of whole foods that will provide you with a similar taste and texture. If you constantly want chips or other salty, crunchy processed foods, eat brown rice cakes or celery and carrot sticks. If you crave creamy foods like chocolate or ice cream, try mixing macadamia butter with raspberries, or eat orange slices topped with plain organic goat milk or soy yogurt.

Use salt sparingly and increase herbs and spices to retrain your taste buds to a healthy sodium intake. Buy sea salt, which contains nourishing trace minerals without the common chemicals, sugar, and aluminum added to standard table salt.

Take a gradual approach to lowering your intake of sweets, refined food, and caffeine.

- Over the course of a few months, cut down on sweet snacks and sweet or caffeinated drinks until you are consuming a minimal amount.
- Drink extra water, herbal tea, fresh vegetable juice, and other unsweetened, replenishing beverages.
- Replace refined sweets with fruits.

Use fruits to sweeten foods the healthy way. Replace food items made with refined sugar or artificial sweeteners with a wide variety of nutritious fruits. Mash up a banana and add it to oatmeal instead of eating cereals sweetened with sugar. Take berries, pears, or the fruit of your choice to work for snacks. Use small quantities of maple syrup or honey when needed. Look for ways to sweeten your life that don't involve food. Say kind, loving words to yourself, and let go of harsh judgment of yourself and others.

Chocolate cravings can signal a depletion of magnesium, common in women with uterine issues. Make sure to eat plenty of magnesium-rich whole foods such as black beans, pumpkin seeds, okra, spinach, Swiss chard, cashews, bananas, brown rice, and halibut. Along with eating an abundance of beans, legumes, vegetables, whole grains, fruits, seeds, and nuts, take magnesium supplements. If you do eat chocolate, buy small amounts of dark chocolate with the least amount of sugar possible.

Stay away from high-fructose corn syrup and other forms of fructose used in refined foods. Fructose is metabolized differently from refined sugar (sucrose). Fructose in processed foods can impair liver health, cause weight gain, and may deplete magnesium from the body. Recently, scientists have found detectable levels of mercury in many popular products containing high-fructose corn syrup. Some companies that produce high-fructose corn syrup use an antiquated manufacturing process that can lead to mercury contamination.

Fat Is Not a Dirty Word

In the last few decades, dietary fats have gotten a bad rap in the West. The message that most of us have received is that fats cause disease, make us unhealthy, and prevent us from having the ideal body. This is only partly true. Certainly, trans fats and high levels of saturated animal fats do contribute to chronic disease, uterine problems, and inflammation. However, there are also fats called essential fatty acids (EFAs) that are necessary for hormonal and cellular balance as well as uterine and ovarian health.

On a regular basis, your body converts carbohydrates into fatty acids, but it cannot produce two types of polyunsaturated EFAs, called alpha-linolenic acid (LNA) and linoleic acid (LA). LNA is an omega-3 fatty acid and LA is an omega-6 fatty acid. These two types of essential fatty acids must come from food. Omega-3 and omega-6 EFAs are eventually converted into prostaglandins, a class of hormone-like chemicals that either encourage or discourage cellular inflammation. Omega-3 EFAs produce series 3 prostaglandins, hormones that are anti-inflammatory and promote uterine relaxation.

The anti-inflammatory omega-3 EFAs can be found in wild cold-water fish, dark leafy greens, seaweed such as dulse, flaxseed and oil, and walnuts. Along with enhancing heart health, brain function, calcium absorption, and healthy skin, omega-3 EFAs can improve fetal development, help prevent postpartum depression, and treat depression during menopause.[7] Omega-3 EFAs also reduce premenstrual breast tenderness, miscarriage, and tumor size, as well as menstrual and endometriosis pain. There is no daily recommended allowance for omega-3 fatty acids, but consuming 1,200 to 4,000 milligrams per day can safely help lessen inflammation.

In my practice I have found that women often see a huge improvement in their uterine health simply by *increasing* their intake of healthy fats. Susana came to see me after having a miscarriage during her first trimester of pregnancy. Like most of my clients, Susana had followed a low-fat diet for many years, thinking she was protecting her heart. However, diets low in healthy fats such as omega-3 EFAs can compromise heart health as well as uterine and ovarian function.

I helped Susana in her grieving process and also encouraged her to make some nutritional changes, including adding more omega-3 fats to her diet. As Susana healed from her loss, I encouraged her to visualize easily conceiving and carrying a healthy pregnancy to term. Eight months later, Susana called to let me know that she was pregnant and had safely made it through her first trimester. Later that year she gave birth to a healthy baby boy.

To support your uterus no matter what stage of life you are in, it is important to consume plenty of omega-3-rich food or supplements. Eat walnuts and a wide variety of dark green leafy vegetables such as kale, spinach, broccoli, and seaweed. Mix ground flaxseeds in smoothies, cereals, stews, and other foods. Keep flaxseeds, flax oil, walnut oil, and any other omega-3-rich oils in the refrigerator and buy in small quantities to prevent spoilage.

Wild cold-water fish such as sardines, herring, mackerel, and wild salmon provide good amounts of omega-3 EFAs when eaten two to three times per week. Smaller fish like sardines generally contain lower mercury levels and are safer to eat on a regular basis than omega-3-rich fish higher up on the food chain, such as swordfish. If you are concerned about mercury levels in fish, you may take fish oil supplements, which have been found to have low mercury levels. You can also increase your consumption of nutrient-rich, high-fiber vegetables and eat ample garlic and cilantro to help clear mercury from your body naturally. Vitamins C and E, the mineral selenium, and supplemental probiotics (discussed later in this chapter) also aid in reducing blood mercury levels.

Like omega-3 fatty acids, omega-6 fatty acids are essential for cellular metabolism. Omega-6 fatty acids are found in most nuts besides walnuts; vegetable oils such as corn, soybean, sunflower, safflower, and sesame; sunflower and sesame seeds; organ meats; and farm-raised fish. Omega-6 fatty acids can be converted to either anti-inflammatory series 1 prostaglandins or inflammatory series 2 prostaglandins. It is important to eat omega-6 fatty acids, but necessary to limit the amounts you consume in proportion to omega-3 EFAs to balance your hormones and heal or prevent uterine problems. Borage oil, evening primrose oil, and black currant oil contain high levels of anti-inflammatory omega-6 EFAs and are thus good for uterine health. To lower your intake of *inflammatory* omega-6 EFAs, decrease your consumption of refined soybean, safflower, sunflower, corn, peanut, or canola oils.

Cook with neutral omega-9 cold-pressed extra-virgin olive oil, but do not let olive oil smoke while cooking. When cooking at high heat, use sesame oil. Instead of eating lowfat or nonfat dressings on salads, use moderate amounts of extra virgin olive oil or walnut oil to help your body absorb the beneficial nutrients from your food. Many antioxidants cannot be absorbed without some amount of healthy fat. Consume fewer inflammatory omega-6 EFAs and more omega-3 EFAs.

It is also essential to eliminate trans fats to support uterine health. Trans fats are often found in margarines, shortening, and many refined foods. Trans fats have been so recently introduced into our diet that your body does not know how to recognize this type of altered fatty acid. These fats have been artificially modified so that the products in which they are used can be stored unrefrigerated for long periods of time. This makes them desirable to industrial food companies, but they can disturb cellular function, block healthy hormone production, block assimilation of healthy fats, and create inflammation and pain in our internal organs, including the uterus. Fortunately, companies are beginning to use fewer trans fats, but they can still be found in many processed foods such as crackers, breads, muffins, chips, cookies, and other manufactured food products. Be sure to read ingredient lists to make sure you are not need-lessly eating trans fats. Eat organic butter, which is much healthier for you in moderate amounts, rather than margarines made with trans fats. Buy trans fat–free products as often as possible or eliminate trans fats completely from your diet to promote uterine wellness.

Reduce your intake of saturated fats from conventionally raised meat and dairy products. The flesh of grain-fed animals, including farm-raised fish such as salmon that are fed corn, has more inflammatory omega-6 EFAs and very little omega-3 EFAs. Meat and dairy from ani-mals that eat grass have higher omega-3 EFAs and lower levels of omega-6 EFAs and are thus not inflammatory. Your body converts convention-ally raised animal fat into inflammatory series 2 prostaglandins that stimulate menstrual and endometriosis cramping, breast tenderness, migraines, and bloating.

High intake of conventionally raised saturated animal fats actually creates inflammation and contributes to uterine problems.

Many nonsteroidal anti-inflammatory drugs (NSAIDs) such as Motrin, Advil, and Nuprin reduce uterine pain and inflammation by inhibiting the production of series 2 prostaglandins. However, you can prevent the production of these inflammatory prostaglandins by changing the balance of the fats you eat instead of having to use medications. By correcting the underlying problem with nutrition, you will support your uterine health and eliminate risks to your stomach, intestines, and kidneys that many women experience from use of NSAIDs.

Eat Smaller Amounts of Animal-Based Foods

Virtually all research shows that rates of benign uterine problems and breast cancer are significantly lower in societies where women eat mostly whole-food, plant-based diets. Meat and dairy raise blood estrogen levels. This is true even for low-fat meats and dairy products because of their high ratios of animal protein. Asian and African women have much lower rates of breast cancer and benign uterine issues than North American or European women. But their rates rise when they immigrate to the United States and start consuming a typical animal-based Western diet.

Women in many non-Western countries have fewer menstrual and menopausal problems because their estrogen levels have consistently been lower from eating mostly plant-based foods, in addition to their reproductive and breast-feeding patterns. Excessive dietary estrogen during the reproductive years can exacerbate menstrual problems, endometriosis, fibroid tumors, and menopausal symptoms. Women in societies that eat plant-based diets do not experience such large declines when their estrogen levels lower at menopause because they were not overly elevated in the first place. Whole-food, plant-based diets consistently create health and can prevent and even reverse chronic uterine disease.

Researchers from the Yale School of Medicine, analyzing more than thirty studies, found that Western women also have much higher rates of hip fracture than women in cultures that eat mostly plant-based calcium and protein.[8] Although it seems counterintuitive to most of us Westerners, who were raised to drink our milk in order to build healthy bones, high levels of animal protein from dairy or meat actually pull calcium from the bones, contribute to calcium loss, and may cause osteoporosis. The more animal protein in food or beverages, the more calcium is required to break down that protein—and that calcium is not made available to our bones. Too much calcium actually blocks the metabolism of vitamin D from sunlight. Vitamin D aids in calcium absorption. Researchers are just realizing how essential environmental vitamin D is in preventing osteoporosis, Alzheimer's, and Parkinson's disease, as well as some kinds of cancer.

Calcium is crucial for uterine health. However, if our animal-based diets play a role in leaching the calcium from our bodies, we risk developing menstrual problems as well as osteoporosis. Dr. Christiane Northrup reveals that up to 50 percent of bone loss actually occurs before menopause for North American women and often starts during the twenties and thirties.[9] It is important to support your body by getting plenty of plant-based calcium in your diet and reducing calcium loss from too many animal proteins, inactivity, smoking, high levels of caffeine, and limited sun exposure. In a twenty-five-year study with 1,800 peri- and postmenopausal women, Californian researchers showed that a whole-foods vegetarian diet can provide enough protein to prevent wrist fracture, a major indicator of osteoporosis.[10]

This does not mean you have to be a vegetarian. In many of the societies with low rates of benign uterine disease, osteoporosis, and breast cancer, people consume some meat, but as a much smaller percentage of their total diet than we typically do in the West. Non-Western women frequently get 10 to 15 percent of their total dietary calories from animal-based foods versus the 70 percent we typically eat.

Consider lowering your percentages of meat, dairy, and eggs and making more plant-based foods the main part of your meal. Instead of eating a big serving of chicken, fish, or meat, divide it up into smaller portions and eat a small amount at dinner and for your next few breakfasts. If you regularly eat with others, share what you previously considered one serving of meat or fish and load up on delicious vegetables and other whole plant-based foods. Increase your intake of plant-based protein such as unsalted nuts, beans, legumes, vegetables, and whole grains.

Some women find that eating organic, hormone-free, animal-based foods eases uterine problems. Pesticides, growth hormones, antibiotics, and other chemicals are stored in the fat cells of animals. Choosing dairy and meat from organically raised animals and those fed on grass rather than grain (including wild fish that can feed on ocean vegetables) will lower your exposure to artificial hormones and other toxins that can negatively affect your endocrine balance. It will also improve the quality of fat you get from animal meats by increasing your ratio of omega-3 EFAs.

If you are experiencing uterine difficulties, try to not eat any dairy for three to six weeks and see if you experience improved health. If that seems too extreme, try consuming only organic dairy and meats or switch to organic goat or sheep milk products, which many people find are easier to digest. Decrease your intake of animal-based foods and increase vegetable-based sources of protein such as unsalted nuts and seeds; beans; legumes such as lentils; green leafy vegetables such as spinach, collards, and kale; and protein-rich whole grains such as quinoa and brown rice, if you can tolerate grains. Eat more vegetable-based calcium such as broccoli, kale, bok choy, turnip greens, green beans, blackstrap molasses, almonds, hazelnuts, sesame seeds, brewer's yeast, prunes, whole grains, and carob flour, and sea vegetables such as nori, kelp, and wakame. Organic, antibiotic-free meat, dairy, and wild fish are more expensive than conventionally raised products, but you will be buying less, which will help with your grocery bill.

Relaxed legal standards in the United States now allow companies to label meat as "natural" as long as animals have not been given hormones or antibiotics within six months of slaughter. Large corporations often give animals growth hormones, antibiotics, and other chemicals for more than a year and still claim that they are hormone free. Ask your grocer to carry meats from farmers who are truly committed to natural standards.

Get Most Nutrients from Food and Use High-Quality Supplements

Obtaining your nutrients, vitamins, and minerals from the food you eat is better than getting them from supplements. However, the typical Western diet and lifestyle frequently deplete the very enzymes and healthy bacteria that are essential for nutritional assimilation. If you lack these necessary enzymes and beneficial intestinal bacteria, you will not be able to get all the nutrients you need from your food alone. Anyone with uterine problems, digestive issues, compromised health, or a history of antibiotic use and yeast infections, as well as people who have eaten substantial amounts of refined foods, can usually benefit from digestive enzymes and probiotics.

Antibiotics, antibiotic products, HRT, hormonal contraceptives, other hormonal medications, chronic stress, and high sugar and refined food consumption strip the digestive system of its healthy bacteria, promoting overgrowth of yeast. Probiotics help restore the healthy bacteria to your body, which in turn strengthens your immune system. This is essential for all women and particularly those with endometriosis, fibroids, yeast infections, constipation, or other elimination problems. Probiotics can safely be used over the long term and are important to use while taking antibiotics and afterward.

As we age, our bodies produce fewer digestive enzymes. Fried, refined, and high-sugar-content foods deplete these precious enzymes even more. Supplementing with digestive enzymes (available at health food stores and online) can improve assimilation of vitamins, minerals, and nutrients from the foods you eat, which can greatly help to heal and prevent a wide range of uterine problems. Explore using enzymes for a month or more and see if you notice improved energy and elimination.

Even though it is best to get your nutrients from whole foods, supplementing with vitamins and minerals can improve uterine health in many cases. Zinc, B vitamins, magnesium, fish oil, vitamin E, vitamin D, and calcium are necessary for healthy hormonal function and can alleviate PMS, menstrual cramping, menopause symptoms, and pain caused by endometriosis. Vitamin B_{12} can only be assimilated well from meat, eggs, and dairy, and vitamin D naturally occurs in fish, meat, eggs, and some cheeses, so vegans will need to make sure they supplement with B_{12} and vitamin D in addition to getting plenty of sunshine. Take a daily multivitamin, but don't rely on supplements for your total vitamin intake. Specific supplement recommendations are discussed in chapters six through eleven.

It is important to eat magnesium- and calcium-rich plant foods and take steps to reduce calcium loss, but it's probably wise to also take a good multimineral supplement that includes magnesium and calcium. Recommended daily calcium intake ranges from 1,000 to 1,500 milligrams per day and varies depending on age, risk factors, and menopausal status. Too much calcium can interfere with the assimilation of other nutrients, so if you have a diet rich in calcium you will want to take smaller amounts of supplemental calcium, or you may not need to supplement with calcium at all. Suggested ratios of calcium to magnesium range from two to one to one to one. Talk to your physician or nutritionist about what is best for you. Calcium citrate is most easily assimilated; calcium carbonate also works well for some women. Caution: if you have a history of kidney stones, do not take calcium supplements unless supervised by your doctor.

Omega-3 oils are rich with vitamin D. Taking cod liver oil is a good way to supplement vitamin D. It is also essential to get vitamin D from the sun. A few times each week, get direct sunlight on your arms and legs for fifteen to twenty minutes before applying sunscreen. If you do not get regular exposure to direct sunlight during winter or rainy seasons, consider taking 2,000 to 3,000 IU of vitamin D_3 daily.

Supplements can be particularly helpful when combined with foods to relieve specific uterine conditions. Adair was a thirty-three-year-old banker I interviewed during my research. The year before we talked, Adair had a Pap test that detected low-grade cervical dysplasia—abnormal cells of the cervix that can lead to cancer. Some cases of low-grade cervical dysplasia may go away on their own, but other types of dysplasia can cause cervical cancer if not discovered and treated. Cervical dysplasia is generally caused by certain strains of the sexually transmitted disease human papilloma virus (HPV) that cause no other symptoms in women, making it essential to have Pap tests regularly. Some researchers suggest that long-term hormonal contraceptives such as the Pill may also result in cervical dysplasia, but there is no definitive answer at this time.

Adair's doctor wanted her to have a conization, surgery that removes a cone-shaped area of cervical tissue. When Adair learned that conization can have side effects such as increased risks of infection and miscarriage, she decided to try a more natural approach. Her doctor did not think that an alternative approach would work, but since cervical cancer does not usually develop immediately from low-grade dysplasia, she was willing to let Adair try.

Adair set up an appointment to meet with a naturopath to see if she could heal these abnormal cells with nutrition, and she and her gynecologist agreed to do another Pap test in three months. If the dysplasia was the same or worse they would set up the conization. If her condition was better, Adair would continue her nutritional approach for another three months to see if she could heal the dysplasia completely.

The naturopath recommended that Adair take a multivitamin daily as well as vitamin B complex, folic acid, vitamin A, cod liver oil, and vitamin C three times each day. She coached Adair to eat more alkaline foods such as vegetables, fruits, miso soup, and chicken while reducing her consumption of acidic foods—particularly red meat, sugar, shellfish, and refined foods.

Adair did not always follow her naturopath's food or supplement directions perfectly, but she made a real effort, and to her delight her condition improved. Within six months the dysplasia had gone away. Her gynecologist wanted to do more screenings every six months for a year and a half to make sure the condition did not return. Adair continued to follow her naturopath's suggestions as well as she could to enhance her health. Consult chapter eleven for further discussion of cervical dysplasia treatments and nutritional strategies to prevent and heal it.

Along with vitamins and nutrients, herbal remedies can be very effective in toning the uterus and correcting some uterine imbalances. Beneficial herbs will be discussed in each chapter in part three. Along with using traditional herbs, flower essences can also help promote uterine wellness. Invented by British physician Dr. Edward Bach in the 1930s, flower essences are like herbal infusions, but they are formulated by using the flowers of plants. Flower essences enhance emotional, spiritual, and physical growth and healing and encourage freedom of expression. Choose essences that relate to your individual condition or energy patterns. Take flower essences three to four times a day by putting a few drops of each essence in a glass of water. Multiple essences can be taken at once.

Transforming Your Relationship with Food

In addition to eating foods that support your uterus, it is important to realize that *how* you eat also significantly influences your uterine health. High percentages of women with endometriosis, fibroids, and other uterine disorders suffer from digestive disorders, irritable bowel syndrome, and basic lack of digestive function that impedes their natural ability to heal. Small changes in your eating habits can help you create a healthier digestive system that will assist in fully absorbing vitamins, enzymes, and nutrients from your food.

Gastrointestinal health is a mirror for overall health. Often when there are uterine imbalances, digestive functions are impaired as well, making it more difficult to heal. Use the strategies suggested here to improve your ingestion, digestion, assimilation, and elimination and create lifelong health.

Make Yourself a Priority: Emotional factors frequently prevent women from implementing healthy eating plans. Guilt, low self-esteem, and negative body image affect women's relationships with food and their health. Feelings of pressure and high stress can cause many women to feel that they cannot even take time to eat or drink water during the day. Christine, an executive in an advertising firm, confessed at our first session that she felt so overwhelmed by her responsibilities that she usually waited until night to eat. She drank as little water as possible during work hours to save the time it takes to later go to the bathroom.

Honor yourself by eating nourishing foods when you are hungry and drinking water throughout your day. Stock up on some healthy snacks and drinks that you can keep at your desk and at home, such as hummus and carrots, or apples and peanut butter, water with lemon, or herbal tea. Having good-tasting nurturing choices on hand is an essential step in eliminating unhealthy habits and cravings without feelings of deprivation.

Become Mindful of *How* You Eat: One factor that is often overlooked in discussions on how to improve nutrition is the importance of chewing your food properly. Eating without chewing well makes it more difficult to digest and assimilate the many different enzymes, nutrients, and vitamins from your food. The whole digestion process actually begins in your *mouth*. By chewing thoroughly, you activate the many digestive enzymes in your mouth and send signals to your entire digestive system that food is on its way to be digested and assimilated, while letting your elimination organs get ready to release any parts of your meal that you do not use. It is important to become aware of your eating patterns and watch how you chew as a first step to gaining more nourishment from your food.

Eat and Cook with Pleasure: Find ways to bring pleasure to every aspect of your meals—including eating your food as well as purchasing or preparing it. If grocery shopping seems like a burden to you, make a weekly grocery shopping or farmers' market date with yourself or a friend. Do something fun either before or afterward. Consider having your groceries delivered or joining a community share program offered by organic farmers in your area.

To make preparing your meals more fun, light candles and turn on some great music. Embrace the simplicity and deliciousness of natural foods, and you will find that cooking can become very easy. Many vegetables are most delicious eaten raw or simply roasted, steamed, or grilled and served plain or with just a little extra virgin olive oil, garlic, lemon, or sea salt. If you are cooking for others, enlist their help with part of the cooking and cleanup, at least some of the time. Share some of your meals with friends, family, or colleagues who inspire you or make you laugh. Savor any opportunity to eat with yourself as an occasion to focus on self-appreciation.

Support All of Your Body's Rhythms: At the other end of the spectrum, women with uterine and other health issues often have problems with elimination. The body's anatomical position is actually hindered while on a toilet, since humans have evolved to squat while eliminating for almost all of our history. Healthy daily elimination patterns can help you restore your health, release toxins, feel better, and ultimately get more nutrients from the foods you eat. Holding your arms in the air or putting your feet on a stool instead of straining while using the toilet can ease your anatomical alignment. Relaxing and breathing slowly and deeply may also help.

You may also find it helpful to do a gentle seasonal nutritional cleanse to support your digestive system. Virtually all cultures throughout human history have refrained from rich foods for certain intervals throughout the year. Strengthen your body by not drinking caffeine or alcohol and not eating refined foods, sugar, red meat, dairy, and other foods that are more difficult to digest for just a few days each season. See the Resources section on page 224 for books that describe nutritional detoxification regimens.

Practice Conscious Eating: For your next few meals, select someplace relaxing and quiet so you can observe how you eat. Take the time to look at your food before you eat so your body can process what it is about to take in. Intend that your meal is going to nourish you completely and that you will digest, assimilate, and eliminate with ease and balance. It is especially helpful to take a few moments to feel gratitude for everything and everybody who made your meal possible—the grocer, the farmer, the worms that irrigate the soil, the earth itself. Give yourself permission to slow down your eating, taste the subtle flavors and textures of your meal, and enjoy every bite.

Use the cognitive restructuring, guided imagery, breathwork, and journaling discussed in chapter three to help you build a positive relationship with food so you can establish lifelong healthy eating patterns and restore or protect your uterine health. Along with incorporating the nutritional strategies in this chapter, make some space in your life to reflect on any eating habits that may be hindering your uterine health.

Addressing these issues is vital for women healing uterine imbalances. For women wanting to prevent uterine health issues, healthy eating is a great way to create wellness at every level. Visualize what you could change in your life to incorporate new healthy ways of eating into your diet. Explore what happens when you strengthen your relationship with food and make food your friend.

Journal on or contemplate the following questions to help you become conscious about your relationship with food:

- What would your relationship with food look and feel like if it really worked?
- What can you celebrate or appreciate right now about your nutrition or relationship with food?
- What difficulties do you encounter in your efforts to improve your eating habits?
- What time restraints, work responsibilities, or family obligations make it difficult for you to maintain a healthy eating plan?
- Are there any thought patterns you have that hinder you in changing your diet?
- Are there any emotions that regularly prevent you from eating in a way that nourishes your health?
- What beliefs about your self-worth would you like to adopt or let go of to be able to nourish yourself with food?
- Are there any people in your life you could ask to help support you in transforming your relationship with food?

Nutritional Changes for Life

Along with deep breathing, stress reduction, healthy movement, and improved posture, increasing your intake of organic vegetables, fruits, and healthy fats while reducing refined and animal-based foods will help you achieve optimal uterine health. Making major lifestyle changes can be difficult, so don't try to transform your eating overnight. Start with whichever of the aspects just discussed feel easiest and most enjoyable to you, such as adding more omega-3 fats or vegetables to your meals or reducing the amount of refined food or sweets you eat. Each month, see whether you can increase your intake of the healthy foods discussed in this chapter while you reduce foods that cause inflammation and uterine distress.

Focus on becoming aware of which foods help you feel your best, and know that you do deserve to feel wonderful—always. If you can't always maintain your ideal diet, please don't stress over it. Remember that increased stress can negatively impact your blood sugar and your uterine health as much as eating inflammatory food.

None of us will always eat perfectly, so have a sense of humor. Every day is new. If you don't eat the way you would like for a few days or weeks, start fresh at your next meal without guilt or shame. Become present to your relationship with food. Release rigidity and punishment and reclaim pleasure.

Relax while you eat, and relax your attitude about what you consume. Enjoy everything you ingest and delight in receiving the bounty of the earth. Don't obsess about food—engage in a wide variety of activities other than eating that provide you with fulfillment, joy, and social connection. Recognize yourself for making an effort to explore new kinds of food, and celebrate your accomplishments as you create better uterine health.

CHAPTER FIVE

Strengthening the Body: Movement, Postural Alignment, and Bodywork

Movement, postural alignment, and self-care techniques that revitalize the body are important components of uterine health. Exercise, proper posture, and self-massage provide more oxygen to the uterus, reduce stress and muscle tension, enhance sexual pleasure, and improve sleep. Aerobic activities increase blood circulation to the uterus, help prevent heart disease, and boost your production of endorphins—the feel-good hormones that relieve pain. Core stability exercises encourage flexibility and healthy spinal alignment, which helps the uterus and surrounding organs remain in optimal position. Strength training and balance exercises assist you in preventing osteoporosis and risk of falls as you age.

Women in societies with low rates of benign uterine health problems are generally much more physically active than women in Western countries. They often engage in activities that align the body and promote proper blood flow to the uterus and other pelvic organs. Many of these societies traditionally employ self-reflexology, massage, or acupressure to prevent uterine pain and inflammation.

You can integrate similar practices into your own life to create optimal uterine health and help alleviate specific uterine problems. All types of movement that feel good to you will support your uterus. Incorporating self-massage, acupressure, or reflexology into your daily regime will help relax your muscles and soothe your nervous system to release pain and promote healing. Becoming mindful of your posture as you walk, sit, and stand will encourage optimal uterine function. Follow the guidelines in this chapter as part of your program to establish uterine wellness. If you have pain, heavy bleeding, or any medical issues, work with your physician to develop an exercise program that will be best for you.

Postural Alignment for Optimal Uterine Health

When I lived in West Africa, I was always amazed at the way women could carry almost anything on their heads. African women would effortlessly transport whatever they wanted—purses, trays of eggs, or large heavy crates—by resting the items on cloths atop their heads. This training starts around two or three years of age for African children, who learn to balance little bowls of water on their heads once they have mastered walking.

I often watched a neighbor's daughter as she acquired this skill. As the water dripped down her face, she learned to relax and extend her spine, enhancing the smoothness of her gait, until one day all the liquid remained in the bowl. In Togo, my friends would regularly try to get me to set my purse on my head because they thought it looked so uncomfortable to constantly have it hanging from my shoulder. I never was able to take more than a few steps without it falling off. However, when I started preparing for natural childbirth, I discovered how the good posture so common with more traditional lifestyles provides women with many more advantages than just being able to easily carry things.

Proper spinal alignment promotes beneficial nerve function and blood flow to the uterus and ovaries, which enhances overall uterine function. Improved posture can help alleviate menstrual cramping and endometriosis pain. It can reduce back pain during pregnancy, correct fetal positioning, and facilitate an easier, quicker birth.

In the West, most of us spend countless hours every week sitting at desks, riding in cars, and relaxing on couches—all activities that can contribute to spinal compression, nerve impairment, and pelvic and uterine misalignment. Our mostly sedentary modern lifestyles cause more than 80 percent of Americans to report back pain each year. The lower back is connected to the uterus by the uterosacral ligaments that help hold the uterus in place. When the back goes out of alignment, the alignment of the pelvis, uterus, and ovaries and the connecting nerve paths and blood flow can be compromised as well. This is because women's bodies have evolved to protect the uterus and any potential offspring it carries.

The uterus is connected to the lower spine, pelvis, hips, and other pelvic organs through a network of strong ligaments and other connective tissue. This network of ligaments helps the uterus stay securely in the pelvis, but also makes the uterus vulnerable to imbalances in the hips and spine. These ligaments affect the function and structure of all pelvic organs, including the uterus, ovaries, fallopian tubes, bladder, and rectum. If out of alignment, they can impair uterine processes.

In my work with clients as well as in my research, I have found that misalignment of the uterus can lead to painful, irregular periods and other uterine imbalances. In severe cases, a tipped or displaced uterus can even affect a woman's ability to become pregnant or carry a pregnancy to term. Fortunately, there are measures you can take to prevent and correct structural imbalances and any corresponding uterine impairment. In my practice, I encourage women to use postural awareness, core strengthening exercises, and, if needed, the help of a physical therapist or chiropractor to help improve pelvic pain, fertility, PMS, and menopausal symptoms.

Women in the traditional societies of Asia and Africa, where rates of menstrual pain, menopause symptoms, and hysterectomies are typically lower, spend much of their time in activities such as walking, farming, and other types of physical work that support uterine alignment. Even when resting, women in developing countries tend to either squat or sit on furniture that encourages upright posture, such as simple benches.

While studying for natural childbirth, I found that midwifery and yoga both advocate squatting as one of the best ways to align the uterus and easily give birth. I remembered all the hours I had spent while doing research in Burkina Faso, West Africa, being amazed that many people seemed to prefer squatting over sitting. Anthropologists are meant to participate as well as observe. Even though I thought I was in pretty good physical shape, I found that it wasn't easy for me to squat for long periods of time as many people do there. During my pregnancy I practiced modified squatting every day. These exercises helped strengthen my uterus and core muscles so I was able to give birth naturally without pain medicine.

You can promote general uterine wellness by becoming more conscious of your posture. Slouching and relaxing back in sofas and chairs causes your pelvis to tip backward, pulling your uterus out of alignment. Sitting, squatting, and standing with your abdomen muscles pulled up and in while you extend your spine helps maintain your pelvis in its natural position. If you spend a lot of time at a desk, sit with your hips and knees at a ninety-degree angle and make sure you have a chair that encourages an upright spine.

Lengthening your spine helps you open your chest and releases your shoulders down your back. In this position you can breathe more easily and your lungs can take in enough oxygen. By expanding your oxygen intake, you boost your immune system and send more nutrients to your muscles and organs, including your uterus.

You can also enhance your uterine health by using Kegel exercises to tone your pelvic floor muscles and help keep your pelvic organs in their proper positions. Kegel exercises involve consciously tightening and releasing the interior muscles of the pelvic floor. They help prevent uterine prolapse and incontinence, relieve some types of pelvic pain, and improve enjoyment during sex.

Uterine prolapse is the major reason for hysterectomy for American women over fifty-five. Women often develop pelvic floor complications after pregnancy and birth that can get worse with age. Incorporate these exercises into your life immediately—do not wait until complications arise. Despite previous concerns, Kegels are now recommended before and during pregnancy to improve labor and postpartum health.

There are several methods you can use to locate the correct pelvic floor muscles you will want to strengthen. You can stand or sit and imagine that a tampon in your vagina is falling out and you need to tighten and raise the vaginal muscles to hold it in. Alternatively, you can squat while you insert a finger into your vagina and squeeze your finger. You can learn to do Kegels by actually stopping the flow of urine while on the toilet, but do not continue this practice after you locate the muscles the first time, as it can create bladder problems. Be sure you engage the muscles in the front part of the pelvic floor within the vagina and not just those near the rectum.

To begin your Kegel practice, either lie on your back with your knees bent and feet flat on the floor, stand, or sit. Initially contract the pelvic muscles for just a few seconds, hold them, and then release them slowly for the same duration. Keep your thighs, buttocks, and abdomen relaxed and still.

Gradually build up the length of time you contract, hold, and release your muscles. Eventually contract, hold, and release your pelvic floor muscles for slow counts of eight a total of forty to fifty times a day, divided up in sets of ten if you like. Also do twenty Kegels daily in which you quickly contract and release the muscles.

I strongly encourage you to incorporate pelvic floor strengthening into your postural alignment. Whenever you focus on your posture, start by pulling your front pelvic floor muscles upward to help engage the deepest level of your abdominal muscles. These will be the vaginal muscles, not those located near the rectum. Several times each day become aware of your front pelvic floor muscles while standing, sitting, or moving. Notice how it feels to take a breath and move them up toward

Once you become comfortable doing Kegels, you can do them anywhere, such as in the shower, standing in line, or at your computer. When done properly, Kegels are not noticeable to others. If you have difficulties contracting the right muscles during Kegels, you can talk to your health care provider or have biofeedback to learn the correct method.

your uterus in a strong, gentle manner while you bring your abdomen in and up, open your chest, and slide your shoulders gently down into your back. Daily practice of Kegel exercises along with regularly engaging your front pelvic floor muscles as part of your healthy posture will help you maintain correct pelvic alignment as you age.

Exercises from Pilates and yoga will help you strengthen your core abdominal and back muscles so that you can more easily develop and maintain proper posture and ensure healthy blood flow to the uterus. Research from Canada shows that core stability training with physiotherapists can help women heal and prevent back and pelvic pain during and after pregnancy.[1] Pilates and yoga both provide good core stability training.

Yoga can help improve menopausal symptoms and decrease PMS. Yoga also offers a wide range of healthy squatting poses that encourage optimal uterine positioning that can be modified for women with physical concerns, including women in the last two trimesters of pregnancy. Whenever you do any exercises that involve abdominal and core strengthening, begin by engaging the front (vaginal) pelvic floor muscles first, pulling them toward your navel as you bring your abdomen up and in toward your spine to build a foundation of strength.

Employ healthy posture while you exercise, stand, move, or sit during your day. Take a few seconds whenever you can to visualize your spine becoming longer and the space between each vertebrae increasing. Imagine there being more room for your uterus and its corresponding nerves and blood vessels. Picture a harmonious flow of energy throughout your whole pelvis and body.

Regular Exercise for Optimal Uterine Health

For nearly all of human history, people have been physically active during most of their waking hours. Our bodies have evolved with this high level of physical activity in mind. Women in traditional societies who regularly engage in a variety of movement throughout their days frequently have low rates of benign uterine problems.

You can build lifelong wellness by developing an exercise routine that includes aerobic activity, core stabilization, flexibility, balance, and strength training. Aerobic exercises can decrease a wide range of menstrual and menopausal symptoms and protect your heart. Strengthening your muscles and core while you build flexibility and balance will help reduce your risk of osteoporosis and falls as you age. Incorporate at least thirty minutes of aerobic activity four times each week, accompanied by strength training, balance exercises, core strengthening, and daily stretching to build flexibility.

Regular walking, running, swimming, cycling, and other kinds of aerobic exercises encourage uterine wellness. Research shows that middle-aged women who participate in aerobic exercise can improve their PMS symptoms considerably.[2] Postmenopausal women can enhance their quality of life and strengthen their bodies with low-impact aerobics.[3] Belly dancing and other dance forms can be a great way to get aerobic exercise while strengthening the mind-body connection and having fun.

Be sure to include interval training in your cardio routine as frequently as possible. Interval training involves repeated periods of high-intensity exercise followed by interludes of low-intensity movement or rest, during which your body recovers. Interval training tones the body more than a regular cardio routine because it constantly challenges the muscles with varied movements. If you repeat similar movements every time you exercise, such as choosing the same program on a cardio machine, your muscles become conditioned to that activity and reach a plateau very quickly. Incorporating interval training helps you reap more benefits from the exercise you do.

There are many different ways to integrate interval training into your workout routine. Walk, run, or cycle up and down a hill, increasing your heart rate on the uphill and giving your body some rest each time you go downhill. You can also use bursts of energy on flat surfaces or in the water to run, walk, cycle, ski, skate, swim, or row as fast as you safely can for intervals of two or three minutes, between which you move more slowly for the same duration of time to let your body recover. You can play sports such as basketball, soccer, ultimate Frisbee, or any game in which periods of intense activity are interspersed with interludes in which you can catch your breath. If you enjoy dancing, alternate songs that inspire faster, then slower moves, or simply use the interval option on any cardio equipment.

Applying this concept of regularly introducing new challenges into other areas of your exercise routine will also bring you more results. When you strength-train, change your routine around each time so your muscles are constantly challenged and introduced to something new. For example, do three sets of each exercise with relatively heavy weights one day, then do six long sets with lighter weights the next time you lift. On other days, use weight training machines and strength exercises that use your body weight, such as push-ups.

If you are currently sedentary, gradually add more movement to your life. Do any kind of physical activity you enjoy. Even ten or twenty minutes a week of sustained movement will help you feel better. Start slowly and build up to exercising at least four days a week for thirty minutes or more. Buy weights to use at home and do at least ten minutes of aerobic movement such as walking or dancing to warm up your muscles before engaging in strength training.

If you have uterine pain, regular stretching for ten to twenty minutes twice a day will help align your posture and decrease pain. High-impact exercise is not recommended for women with endometriosis or other

Consider doing activities that combine multiple benefits, such as strength building and aerobic movements or core stabilization with flexibility and balance training. Martial arts such as aikido and judo, gymnastics, and some forms of yoga provide aerobic activity while strengthening the body and enhancing core stability, balance, and flexibility. Horseback riding, rowing, and tennis help build strength and aerobic capacity.

severe pelvic pain. Restorative yoga and other forms of gentle exercises such as tai chi, qi gong, Alexander Technique, Feldenkrais Method, or Rosen Method Movement are especially beneficial for women experiencing pain, heavy menstrual bleeding, or other challenging symptoms that might make some forms of high-impact aerobic exercise uncomfortable. Alexander and Feldenkrais approaches involve simple exercises that help expand posture, ease pain, and create more freedom of movement. Tai chi and qi gong offer specific series of movements that help balance the body's energy and strengthen core muscles. The Nia Technique blends all of these forms with dance to create a mind-body movement form that many women enjoy. Rosen Method Movement combines a series of physical therapy exercises to align the body, increase range of motion, facilitate emotional expression, and release pain.

If you have been sedentary for a long time or feel depleted or shut down emotionally, a tai chi, qi gong, Alexander Technique, Feldenkrais Method, Nia, or Rosen Method Movement class or DVD may offer a wonderful way to support your uterine health by helping you become more active and improving your posture. Integrating simple yogic balance poses into your regular exercise routine is helpful for women at every fitness level. Doing balance poses several days a week can help prevent fractures as you age. If you ever feel like you need assistance, practice balance poses near a wall and ask your instructor for other modifications to avoid injury. Always stretch after exercise to relax your muscles and improve flexibility.

If you have pain from endometriosis, fibroids, or menstruation that sometimes feels too severe to allow you to exercise, consult with a physical therapist or qualified yoga instructor to develop stretches that you can do daily. Research shows that easy stretches or restorative yoga will relax and extend tight pelvic muscles and decrease pelvic pain.[4] Work up to doing thirty minutes of low-impact aerobic exercise at least three days a week, combined with strength training, daily yoga, stretching, or other gentle mind-body techniques that help you balance your energy and improve your posture.

Self-Care Bodywork Techniques

In my early twenties I stayed with a family in Chongqing, a large city in southwestern China. Each night after dinner the family would partake in a beautiful foot-washing ritual. Instead of scattering to their various rooms, my hosts would sit together and take turns washing and massaging each person's feet as well as the ankles and calves of the women in the family.

Through my friend's interpretation, her grandmother told me that it is extremely important for people to have the pressure points of their feet rubbed each night to strengthen the internal organs and balance the body. She shared that including women's ankles and calves in the massage helps maintain uterine function. As I sat in the sparse Chinese apartment, I was transported back to my childhood. I recalled visiting my great-aunt in a rural part of the Arkansas Ozarks as she taught me reflexology, the practice of stimulating certain areas of the feet, hands, or ears to strengthen the nervous system and improve physiological function.

Even though rural Arkansas and urban China may seem light years apart, both of these experiences illustrate how women in traditional cultures have passed on knowledge about uterine wellness for thousands of years. For millennia, women have used acupressure, reflexology, and self-massage to decrease pain during pregnancy and birth, regulate menstrual cycles, and prevent menopausal symptoms. Anthropologists report that these "low-tech" methods are still commonly used in many communities in Latin America, Asia, and Africa. These modalities work by applying pressure to certain points on the body to revitalize organs, improve blood circulation, release endorphins, enhance lymphatic and energy flow, and decrease muscle and connective tissue pain.

I encourage you to use self-acupressure, reflexology, or massage for a few minutes each day to promote uterine wellness and decrease problematic symptoms. Do these techniques in a calm environment where you can focus your entire awareness on healing your body. Breathe deeply and slowly and set an intention that your actions will enhance or restore your uterine health. Feel free to add small amounts of essential oils to massage oil during self-massage, reflexology, or acupressure to soothe your nervous system and enrich your experience. Like most mind-body therapies, these modalities will begin to restore and relax your body immediately, but they must be practiced regularly over many months, combined with nourishing nutrition and stress-reduction techniques, to heal chronic uterine conditions. I recommend you make whichever of these practices appeal to you a part of your lifelong self-care regime.

You can strengthen your uterine health and relieve pain by massaging your feet, ankles, calves, abdomen, neck, and head regularly. Wear loose clothing or undress for your massage. Use massage oil on bare skin. Sit upright in a chair or lie on your back with your knees bent so you can easily reach your feet.

Start your massage with your feet and calves. Begin with your left foot by making long gentle strokes from your toes to your ankle, then up your calf, to relax your body. Return to the toes of your left foot. Rub the sides, top, and bottom of each toe. Gently stretch your toes. Massage the bottom and top of your left foot from the ball to the ankle, making a circular motion with your fingers. Use whatever amount of pressure feels good to you.

Stroke your left ankle with your thumb and fingers using firm, but comfortable pressure. Glide your hands up and down the front, back, and sides of your left calf to warm up your leg. Make circular motions using your thumb or fingers from the base of your left calf to your knee. Do this massage technique over your entire left calf. Repeat the massage on your right foot, ankle, and calf.

Gently glide the palm of either hand in clockwise circles over your abdomen. Stroke your belly like this for a minute or more, using the entire surface of your hand.

Close your eyes during the neck and head portion of your massage. Use both hands to massage the sides, front, and back of your neck, working from your collarbone and moving up to your head.

Begin your head massage by lightly caressing your face from your chin to your forehead with the pads of your fingers, avoiding the soft tissue near your eyes. Use circular strokes on your temples and all over the top of your skull. Knead the sides of your head around your ears, using somewhat firmer pressure if it feels good. Start at the base of the back of your head, making tiny circles with each finger while you continue the massage toward the top of the head. Finish by lightly gliding your fingers along your jaw from each ear to your chin. Take a few deep breaths before you open your eyes.

Daily foot, calf, belly, neck, and head massage for five to ten minutes can be very effective in reducing uterine pain, easing PMS, headaches, insomnia, or hot flashes and night sweats during menopause. Massage from either yourself or another person can also help circulation and decrease pain during pregnancy, birth, and postpartum. It is an excellent way to boost your immune system and prevent uterine imbalances from occurring.

Regularly performing the simple reflexology and acupressure techniques described next will also help support uterine function. When stimulating these regions, apply firm but comfortable pressure with the pads of your thumbs or fingers. Activate each area as specified for one to two minutes once a day to enhance uterine wellness or three to five minutes twice a day to help heal uterine imbalances. The spots you are looking for may be tender. Use firm pressure, but never so much force that you produce pain. Breathe and relax and enjoy any changes you feel in your body.

For reflexology, stand next to a chair and place your right foot in the seat of the chair with your knee bent. Bend down so your hand can easily reach your foot. With your thumb, apply firm pressure above your heel on the inside of the ankle. Stroke with your thumb up and down in this area on the inner side of your foot, just above the heel and behind the large ankle bone. Then move your thumb to the same area on the outer side of your foot and use the same up-and-down stroke. Repeat on your left foot. Regularly massaging these areas strengthens uterine and ovarian function.

For acupressure, put your right foot back on the chair. Place your index finger on the top of your right foot between your big and second toes to locate the LV 3 (Liver 3) point. Make circular strokes with your finger in between the bones of your big and second toes, gently massaging this point to help support your liver and regulate your estrogen levels. The next point, SP 6 (Spleen 6), can be found four finger widths above your inner ankle near the back of your inner calf. Simply press on Spleen 6. Stimulating this point is very helpful for uterine health, but never activate this point during pregnancy or if you think you might be pregnant, as it acts to expel the fetus. Use a gentle circular massage on SP 10 (Spleen 10), which is located right above your knee on the inside of your thigh. If you straighten and flex your leg you will find this point at the bottom of your quadriceps muscle where it bulges out directly above your kneecap. Switch legs and use the same techniques on the same points on your left foot and leg. If you are pregnant, check with an acupuncturist before you do any self-acupressure.

Thousands of women have also successfully used self-care techniques such as the Emotional Freedom Technique (EFT) or Reiki to ease uterine problems. EFT is an easy-to-learn acupressure method that reduces pain and releases trapped emotions. EFT involves a series of light tapping on areas of the body exhibiting pain. You can learn about EFT through the free website www.emofree.com. Reiki is a Japanese hands-on energy healing technique used throughout the world to decrease pain and promote healing and relaxation. Like acupuncture and acupressure, Reiki is used in many hospitals in the United States to speed recovery

In addition to your hands, you can use tennis balls to activate reflexology or acupressure points or various massage tools to make self-massage even easier. This may be particularly helpful if you have hand pain or arthritis. There are also exercise programs, such as the Myofascial Energetic Length Technique (MELT) Method and Yamuna Body Rolling, that use rollers and balls to stimulate pressure points and reduce chronic pain.

from surgery and chemotherapy and reduce patient pain without the side effects of drugs. You can train to do Reiki on yourself and others in just one weekend. Additionally, acupuncturists consider qi gong practice an excellent way to open up your energy pathways and heal your body.

Acupressure, reflexology, massage, EFT, and Reiki are easy to perform on yourself. However, if you would like more assistance, see a practitioner for any of these modalities. Acupuncture is effective at alleviating a wide range of uterine imbalances, such as hot flashes, PMS, and pelvic pain. A few sessions of massage, acupressure, acupuncture, or Reiki from a trained therapist have been demonstrated to promote uterine healing and can be a great noninvasive way to improve PMS, hot flashes, or pain from endometriosis and fibroids. Gentle forms of energy work such as Reiki and acupressure from a trained practitioner with experience working with women's healing can be particularly beneficial for women who have experienced sexual trauma or abuse.

Women experiencing chronic uterine and pelvic pain may also benefit from the support of a physical therapist or chiropractor to help heal muscle and nerve damage while they bring their bodies into alignment and increase activity levels. Chiropractic treatments combining spinal adjustments and soft tissue therapy improved PMS symptoms for women in Australia.[5] In the United States, physical therapy techniques have been shown to reduce endometriosis and pelvic pain.[6] In some cases they can also reverse infertility for women with tubal obstructions and pelvic scarring, including those with endometriosis.

I have interviewed a number of women who feel that chiropractic treatments, physical therapy, or other types of manual bodywork have helped them heal PMS, hot flashes, and infertility. If you have fibroids, endometriosis, debilitating menstrual pain, or menopausal symptoms, consider seeing a physical therapist for a complete musculoskeletal evaluation or having chiropractic treatments. I refer clients who are concerned about the physicality of traditional chiropractic adjustments to chiropractors who restore spinal structure and nervous system function by balancing the body's energy. Chiropractors who use Network, Bio

Energetic Synchronization Technique (BEST), or biocranial techniques align the spine and the nerves throughout the body with gentle manipulations that do not involve forceful work on the spine or joints.

In the United States, a few forms of complementary healing such as acupuncture are beginning to be covered by some insurance plans, but in most instances you will have to pay out of pocket for mind-body treatments. This can seem like a big expense. However, making this investment in your health and healing may actually save you money in the long run. Often holistic health treatments are less expensive than co-pays for surgery, missed work, some prescription medicines commonly used for uterine issues, and most infertility treatments. There are of course no guaranteed results, but for many women investing in treatments with a qualified healer is well worth it.

Honor Your Body

Women who live in societies that encourage more active lifestyles, good posture, and self-care bodywork techniques frequently have fewer benign uterine difficulties than those of us who live in industrialized societies. Make time every day for movement, postural awareness, and easy-to-use self-care techniques to enhance your uterine health. Along with helping to prevent and heal uterine disorders, regular exercise, structural alignment, and self-care bodywork will soothe your nervous system, balance hormones, accelerate healing, deepen your sleep, improve your immune system, and strengthen your body as you age.

Make these activities part of your daily routine and social life. Stand up from your computer twice an hour to stretch and lengthen your spine. Balance on one foot while you brush your teeth or wait for the bus. Do Kegel exercises while you sit at your desk or talk on the phone. Go for walks or play a friendly game of sports with your family or friends. Take a Reiki class with someone you know or do a massage swap with a friend or partner.

If you do not currently engage in exercise and other techniques discussed in this chapter, be gentle with yourself as you embark on transforming your lifestyle. Keep a journal of the activities you do, including exercise, self-massage, reflexology, or acupressure. Along with recording the date of the event, write down how you feel after each activity and observe how this may change over time. Start with adding in activities you enjoy that feel good. Focus on your success as you release stress and pressure from your life.

PART THREE

Uterine Health Conditions

CHAPTER SIX

Menstruation

The menstrual cycle consists of a series of physiological changes in the uterus, ovaries, and endocrine system that take place from the beginning of one menstrual flow to the start of the next. Each menstrual cycle begins with menstruation—the periodic shedding of the uterine lining. Once menstruation is completed, the endometrium, or uterine lining, begins to thicken and the ovaries prepare eggs for ovulation—the release of a mature egg into the fallopian tube. During this time estrogen levels increase and peak right before ovulation. Ovulation usually occurs on day fourteen or fifteen of the menstrual cycle, causing progesterone levels to rise and the uterus to relax and produce a nutrient-rich home for the potential embryo. If pregnancy does not take place within ten to twelve days following ovulation, a drop in progesterone and estrogen causes the endometrium to break down and once again menstruation occurs.

During this cyclical hormonal dance, millions of Western women experience pain, bloating, headaches, anxiety, excessive bleeding, and other symptoms that create havoc in their lives. The outlook on menstruation in the United States can be summed up by just a few of the terms that have been used over the years to describe it: the curse, the red plague, the bloody scourge, and the weeping womb.

Throughout most of human history, women experienced later ages of menarche, more pregnancies, and significantly longer time spent breast-feeding. These reproductive health patterns (accompanied by more physical lifestyles and lower protein diets) resulted in dramatically fewer menstrual periods during the average woman's lifespan. Today, in developing countries across the globe, women's dietary, lifestyle, childbirth, and breast-feeding patterns still more closely reflect those of our ancestors. In many of these societies women normally menstruate as little as four times per year, on average.

Millions of indigenous South American, South Asian, or African women may menstruate only one hundred times during their lives. In contrast, their Western counterparts will typically start menarche earlier, have very few children, breast-feed for shorter periods, and eat diets rich in calories, estrogen, and meat protein. As a result, the average Western woman can expect to experience four times as many menstrual periods—more than four hundred of them between menarche and menopause. This relatively sudden lifestyle shift—in evolutionary terms—has given Western women's bodies very little time to adjust to these massive changes.

Some women's health experts propose to correct this pattern by artificially inhibiting women's menstrual cycles through the use of synthetic hormones. Unfortunately, this strategy rarely delivers lifelong wellness. In fact, long-term suppression of menstruation through artificial means generally strains the liver and creates additional health problems. Instead, follow the Optimal Uterine Health Plan (part two) and the integrative suggestions in this chapter to support your body, heal underlying imbalances, and develop uterine and menstrual wellness.

Biomedical Approaches to Menstruation

Conventional medicine classifies normal menstruation as cyclical uterine bleeding that occurs for a four- to seven-day period every twenty-four to thirty-five days. Uterine bleeding is considered abnormal if it is infrequent (oligomenorrhea), occurs more often than every twenty-one days (polymenorrhea), happens at irregular intervals (metrorrhagia), lasts longer than seven days and is so heavy that you have to change your tampon or pad more often than every two hours (menorrhagia), is excessive and irregular (menometrorrhagia), occurs after sex (postcoital bleeding), is absent during the reproductive years (amenorrhea), occurs after menopause, or has no apparent cause (dysfunctional uterine bleeding).

Hormone imbalances, nonuterine diseases, infections, miscarriage, ectopic pregnancies, fibroid tumors, uterine polyps, endometrial hyperplasia, endocrine disorders, malignancies, and precancerous conditions can cause abnormal uterine bleeding. Most abnormal uterine bleeding is noncancerous, but if you experience irregular uterine bleeding it is important to consult your health care provider to confirm diagnosis. In many cases, your physician may perform an endometrial biopsy—a procedure used to examine a small amount of the uterine lining, to make sure that any irregular bleeding is not caused by uterine cancer.

Depending on the cause of benign abnormal uterine bleeding, gynecologists will generally prescribe hormonal medications, hormonal contraceptives, or nonsteroidal anti-inflammatory drugs (NSAIDs) to regulate menstruation. To control heavy bleeding that does not respond to medication, physicians may recommend surgical procedures. Dilation and curettage (D & C) removes uterine tissue to temporarily prevent bleeding and provide a diagnostic sample. Endometrial ablation destroys and scars the uterine lining to permanently stop menstruation. In the case of malignancies and serious conditions, a hysterectomy may be suggested. Hysterectomies should be a last-resort procedure for benign uterine problems. If your physician recommends a hysterectomy for menstrual problems with no apparent cause, get a second opinion.

Dysmenorrhea, or menstrual cramps, affects more than 50 percent of all menstruating women in the West. Dysmenorrhea is categorized as either primary, when pelvic pain results from the menstrual cycle and occurs in the absence of other pelvic disease, or secondary, when it is caused by conditions such as endometriosis. Medical practitioners usually prescribe hormonal contraceptives or NSAIDs to decrease the inflammatory prostaglandin hormones that cause cramps.

If your cramps are severe, last throughout your period, and worsen as you age, and your menstrual flow is heavy, consult your doctor to see if you have adenomyosis, a condition in which the cells of the uterine lining grow into the muscular walls of the uterus. Adenomyosis usually occurs after women have had children; it may be initiated by cesarean section or other uterine surgery, but currently the cause is not known for certain. Most physicians will use the same treatment protocol for cramps. If unsuccessful, many doctors will suggest hysterectomy. Adenomyosis will go away after menopause when estrogen levels lower. Use the self-help guidelines in the endometriosis chapter to balance your estrogen levels and attempt to alleviate symptoms of adenomyosis naturally.

Premenstrual syndrome (PMS) is a medical category of more than one hundred symptoms thought to be related to the hormonal changes that occur between ovulation and menstruation—symptoms such as anxiety, depression, pain, cramps, mood swings, and anger. Most American women report some sort of physiological and emotional changes during the premenstrual phase. PMS affects 40 to 50 percent of menstruating women, who find that these changes cyclically create challenges in their daily lives and then go away before or shortly after their periods begin. Premenstrual dysphoric disorder (PMDD) is considered a more severe form of PMS that impairs the lives of approximately 3 to 5 percent of menstruating women. Some medical experts believe that PMDD may be more of a psychiatric condition and may be a separate disorder from PMS. Causes of PMS or PMDD are not known for certain, and no diagnostic tests are available. Hormonal contraceptives, antidepressants, diuretics, and cognitive therapy are used to treat symptoms.

Menstrual irregularities, premenstrual discomfort, and cramps can impair women's lives and pose serious health risks such as anemia in the case of heavy bleeding. Medications such as hormonal treatments, NSAIDs, antidepressants, and hormonal contraceptives can help reduce PMS symptoms and restore menstrual patterns, and unlike most surgeries, they are less invasive and reversible. However, they rarely correct underlying imbalances, and they can cause other health problems if taken for prolonged periods. If you choose medication to regulate menstruation or prevent cramps or PMS symptoms, implement holistic strategies to support your body while on medication and create mind-body wellness. Use the cognitive restructuring, breathing, visualization, and anti-inflammatory nutrition guidelines in this book to eventually taper off medication and remain symptom-free, or make nutritional and stress-reduction changes your first response to alleviate inflammation, irregular menses, cramps, and PMS naturally.

Continue to have yearly pelvic exams and regular Pap tests as recommended by your doctor to detect cervical abnormalities early and prevent cervical cancer. Women over thirty without new or multiple partners who have had three consecutive clear Pap tests may be advised to only repeat Pap tests every two to three years. Talk to your doctor about how often you need Pap tests and have yearly gynecologic examinations. Always consult your health care provider if you experience further abnormal menstruation to rule out uterine cancer.

Talking with Your Doctor

Track any symptoms you have during your menstrual cycles and share the results you find with your care provider to help him or her understand your situation more fully. Be sure to tell your physician how frequently and heavily or lightly you bleed during menstruation, including the kind of protection you use—such as super or regular tampon or type of pad—and how often you need to change your protection. Even if discussing this information seems embarrassing to you, it is crucial that you record it and share it with your care provider so that he or she can help you.

Holistic Approaches to Menstruation

In holistic health traditions, menstruation is welcomed as a positive, natural part of a woman's life. Problems are thought to arise when societies do not honor female power or when women feel unable to adequately care for themselves or express their energies freely. Rather than practicing symptom management, integrative medicine seeks to heal the underlying conditions causing premenstrual and menstrual imbalances. Focusing on mind-body dynamics, complementary modalities help women revitalize their uterine, endocrine, and menstrual health through whole-foods nutrition, exercise, stress reduction, energy restoration, and hormonal balance.

Nutrition, Supplements, and Herbs

A nourishing diet is essential for menstrual health. A balanced intake of fresh vegetables, fruits, and essential fatty acids (EFAs), accompanied by the reduction of refined foods, refined sweets, trans fats, and saturated fats, is vital to diminishing the inflammation that causes menstrual irregularities, cramps, heavy flow, and PMS symptoms. Follow the recommendations in chapter four and, as much as possible, eliminate caffeine, alcohol, and processed foods from your diet.

Women who experience PMS have consistently been found to have diets much higher in refined foods, sugar, dairy, and salt, and deficient in essential nutrients. Take time to gradually change the foods you eat, week by week, so you can experiment to find enjoyable, healthy alternatives. Replace refined grains with whole grains: for example, have quinoa or other whole grains instead of pasta for lunch or dinner or eat brown rice cakes instead of crackers, chips, or bread. Eat fewer processed foods in general and add in more red, green, orange, and yellow vegetable dishes to your meals. If you now eat meat every day, try eating organic tofu instead of meat once a week. Gradually replace refined sweets with fruit. Use anti-inflammatory ginger abundantly.

Increase omega-3 EFAs with daily intake of fish oil, flax oil, freshly ground flaxseeds, hemp seeds, and walnuts while you decrease meat and reduce or eliminate dairy. Flax reduces inflammation and regulates menstrual cycles. Mix ground flaxseeds into your cereals, soups, or smoothies, and eat at least two tablespoons per day. Put hemp seeds on salads. If you do like animal foods, choose organically raised meat and dairy fed grass rather than corn and eat wild cold-water fish such as sardines, mackerel, or halibut. To ease PMS, boost your production of anti-inflammatory prostaglandins by supplementing with evening primrose oil, black currant oil, and borage oil, which are all rich in gamma linolenic acid (GLA). Use cold-pressed oils as often as possible.

Get plenty of dietary calcium from plant-based sources. A 2005 study in the *Archives of Internal Medicine* confirms that increased calcium and vitamin D from food can prevent the development of PMS and menstrual problems.[1] Women with PMS and PMDD are frequently deficient in vitamin D, magnesium, and calcium. Magnesium relaxes muscle tissue, decreases menstrual cramps, strengthens bones, and helps the liver metabolize estrogen. Industrial agriculture has depleted magnesium from soils, making it more difficult to obtain sufficient dietary magnesium.

Calcium deficiency during the reproductive years may result in more vasomotor symptoms at menopause, such as hot flashes, as well as osteoporosis. To support your lifelong health, eat plenty of organic calcium- and magnesium-rich foods. Take a multimineral and a multivitamin, and expose large parts of your skin to direct outdoor sunlight without sunscreen twice a day for fifteen minutes to get ample vitamin D. If you have heavy menstrual flow, eat iron-rich plant foods such as blackstrap molasses, wheat germ, and brewer's yeast to prevent anemia; take iron supplements if needed. Make sure you get sufficient zinc, selenium, B vitamins, and vitamins A, C, and E. Even if you do not want to make major changes in your eating habits, supplement with the following to significantly reduce pain, regulate flow, and decrease PMS symptoms:

- B vitamins, including B_6
- Evening primrose oil
- Fish oil
- Ground flaxseed or flax oil
- Magnesium
- Vitamin E
- Zinc

Traditional Chinese medicine attributes PMS and menstrual irregu-larities to liver dysfunction. A variety of herbs can assist your liver and balance the menstrual cycle. To strengthen your liver, take dandelion, milk thistle, yellow dock, nettle leaf, and burdock root. To tone the uterus and ease menstrual problems—including cramps, PMS, and irregular kinds of uterine bleeding—use raspberry leaf, wild yam, and chaste tree. Naturopath Tori Hudson recommends using yarrow, squaw vine, vitex, and mugwort to promote menstrual flow for women with infrequent or absent menstruation and yarrow, lady's mantle, cranesbill, and shep-herd's purse to reduce heavy flow.[2]

Exercise and Bodywork

Women who exercise regularly report fewer problems with premen-strual pain, mood, and concentration.[3] Regular movement—such as walking, running, dancing, yoga, and stretching—can improve men-strual health by increasing the blood flow to the uterus and pelvic organs. Aerobic activities help you produce endorphins—natural feel-good hormones that can alleviate cramping and other menstrual pain. A half hour of aerobic exercise four days a week, accompanied with weight training, yoga, or Pilates, will help you feel better. If you have heavy menstrual flow and you feel tired, weak, or short of breath during exer-cise, see your doctor immediately to determine whether you are anemic. If you have amenorrhea, partake in gentle exercise and do not exercise or train excessively.

Practicing yoga or stretching for ten minutes each day will promote spinal and pelvic alignment and relax tight muscles in the back and pel-vis. Yoga positions such as forward bend (*paschimotanasana*), cobra (*bhujangasana*), bow (*dhanurasana*), cat (*bidalasana*), shoulder stand (*sarvangasana*), fish (*matsyasana*), and revolved triangle (*parivrtta triko-nasana*) can help regulate menstruation and decrease cramps, backaches, and headaches. If you have severe back or neck pain, avoid the bow pose, shoulder stand, and cat pose. Always follow shoulder stand with fish pose to balance the front and back of the body. Do not do shoulder stand, other yogic inversions, or strenuous backbends while menstruating. Instead of inversions, lie on your back with your legs up resting on the wall (*viparita karani*) and support yourself in backbends or strenuous standing poses during your period. Begin your yoga postures by taking a few deep breaths while sitting in a crossed-legs pose (*sukhasana*) to help lengthen your spine. End by lying down and breathing deeply in corpse pose (*savasana*) to help you relax fully.

Use the self-massage and basic acupressure and reflexology directions in chapter five to promote overall menstrual health. If you need additional assistance, seek help from a chiropractor, acupuncturist, or acupressure practitioner to help strengthen your uterus, liver, endocrine and nervous systems and diminish menstrual symptoms naturally.

Conscious Breathing

In chapter one, I explain that the chakra framework is an important aspect of mind-body medicine. In Hindu philosophy, the chakras are powerful energy centers that influence health and wellness in the body. The seven main chakras extend from the tailbone to the crown of the head and relate to the various organs located in each energy center, or "wheel of light." The uterus sits in the second chakra. You can use this breathing exercise to strengthen your second chakra, uterus, ovaries, and digestive tract and to make menstruation easier.

Second Chakra Breathing Exercise: Following the guidelines for uterine breathing in chapter three, either sit or lie down in a safe, quiet setting. Release tension from each area of your body as you start to take full breaths. Allow your breath to expand as you focus your awareness on your lower abdomen area. Breathe deeply into your lower belly and back, including the area in the center of your body between your back and abdomen. With every breath, relax more fully.

Breathe nourishing energy into the second chakra area between your lower abdomen and back. Feel a soft warmth in this area or envision a beautiful orange glow emerging throughout your second chakra. Expand your breath and the warmth, energy, or light that it brings to all of the organs, muscles, and tissues in your lower abdomen and back.

Continue breathing and know or intend that your whole second chakra area is attracting amazing power, health, and vitality. Trust that these qualities—or others, such as love, light, and creativity—are flowing from the universe into your whole second chakra with every inhalation. Believe that every cell in your lower back and lower abdomen is filling with these healing qualities as you easily release guilt, anger, shame, fear, and disease with every exhalation. Continue to breathe and feel this energy as long as you would like. Know that your second chakra as well as your menstrual cycle and whole body are strengthening and revitalizing.

Cognitive Restructuring

Research shows that cognitive restructuring helps decrease PMS.[4] It can also reduce stress, which makes integrating nutritional and exercise changes easier. Use the guidelines in chapter three to journal about menstruation. You may want to begin your journaling process by writing about how you would like your menstrual cycle to be in your life. Imagine your ideal experience and write about what it would feel like if your menstrual cycle could be really healthy and balanced. Next, journal about any challenges your menstrual cycle creates and what steps you could take to lessen these challenges. Write about any positive aspects that you feel menstruation brings to your life.

Also explore if you have any attitudes about menstruation that may increase the stress in your life. In my research I found that women who reported numerous physical problems with their cycles frequently held more negative attitudes about menstruation. Several women that I interviewed described how their problems with menstruation have negatively affected their identity as women because they felt that it is unfair for women to have to carry such burdens. Use your journaling to examine how your attitudes about menstruation affect your relationship with your body, your stress levels during your cycle, or your identity as a woman. Consider whether you possess any negative views about your body, such as disdain for your period, and if so, whether transforming your beliefs about menstruation could help you improve your uterine health.

Write about what it would be like if your society honored menstruation and provided women with extra space and nourishment during the menstrual process. Journal on ways you can increase self-care and creative expression during menstruation to help make your process easier and more enjoyable. Create a ritual to honor yourself as a menstruating woman to help enhance the energy around menstruation in your life.

Visualization

Natasha came to see me about painful periods and severe PMS. A talented young lawyer in Washington, D.C., Natasha experienced mood swings every month before her period that made her frustrated at work and angry at her coworkers. In our initial session, I asked Natasha to keep a record, over the next two months, of exactly when in her cycle she had pain, cramping, bloating, mood swings, anger, or difficulties relating to others. In the meantime, Natasha and I met twice a month, helping her lower stress, transform disempowering beliefs, and develop nutritional support to strengthen her uterus and reduce inflammation.

Over time, the nutrition, cognitive restructuring, and stress-reduction changes relieved most of Natasha's symptoms. However, she still experienced intense frustration that made relating to others difficult during the premenstrual phase, so I suggested that we use physiological imagery to promote proper uterine function. Natasha initially expressed doubts that visualization could help something that had seemed so overpowering and out of control for most of her adult life. I explained that physiological imagery is used extensively in hospital settings and has been consistently shown to improve health outcomes, even with people experiencing advanced, debilitating diseases. I also assured Natasha that other clients who initially expressed similar hesitancy had found imagery to be a very effective tool to regulate cycles and decrease menstrual problems. Natasha agreed to give imagery a try.

At our subsequent appointment, we determined that Natasha experienced frustration each month for two or three days right before she started her period. Her anger increased during the time when the endometrial tissue that covers the uterine wall in order to implant the ovum begins to break down in order to be shed in menstruation, since no pregnancy has occurred. I pointed out that perhaps Natasha felt anxiety about starting her period, which could contribute to her feeling more anxious during this time. When I mentioned that the endometrium is a mucous membrane layer of cells that produce some mucus during the second half of the menstrual cycle, Natasha said that it grossed her out that there would be mucus in her uterus. She told me she had always been a little put off by everything that happened "down there." She never wanted to think about it, which is why she had been so uncomfortable regarding the visualization.

The idea of her uterus producing and expelling small amounts of mucus every month was hard for her to imagine—Natasha considered mucus clingy and gross, and she couldn't picture it shedding easily. I raised the idea that viewing this process as difficult, disgusting, and negative was perhaps part of the problem. I mentioned that other organs, like the lungs, also produce mucus and suggested that seeing this process as beautiful, natural, and easy might help her body function better.

Natasha had a few laughs, took a deep breath, and closed her eyes. I guided her to sense the endometrium easily breaking down and leaving her body as balanced, healthy menstrual flow. I suggested that she imagine white light flowing into her uterus filling the space where the endometrial tissue was. At the end of our session, Natasha told me that when she pictured the white light filling her uterus, she felt a sense of unexpected calm come over her. She laughed and said that she never thought she would be doing something quite so strange, but if it worked, it would be worth it.

I asked Natasha to do this guided imagery daily for the next six weeks and then as often as she could on a regular basis. We agreed that she would practice this visualization three times a day during the week before her period. We continued our work together to help her get in touch with her anger and the beliefs and life patterns that caused it. A few weeks later, Natasha called me, saying she could not believe it. She had felt great and was completely relaxed during what was normally her PMS week. She told me that it was much easier for her to let go and disengage from frustrating situations to give herself a chance to breathe and get some perspective on how best to proceed. She felt much more stable; some of her coworkers had even remarked on her calmness.

Physiological imagery can be very healing if used regularly. It requires a basic understanding of the biological processes involved, so research the specific part of the menstrual process you would like to improve and speak to your health care provider if you have any questions. If you experience internal resistance or hesitation about visualizing your menstrual cycle, use the exercises in the previous section on cognitive restructuring to embark on a new way of viewing your body. For more physiological guided imagery scripts, consult the books listed in the Resources section (page 221). If physiological imagery does not appeal to you, imagine yourself feeling balanced and healthy during your entire menstrual cycle and use the symbolic visualizations in chapter three as well as the Endocrine Gland Visualization in chapter ten. The most important aspect of visualization is to evoke pleasure, relaxation, and joy in your body and mind. Choose imagery that assists you in doing that to the fullest.

A Purification Process

The mind-body practices just described create ease during your menstrual cycle by strengthening your uterus, endocrine system, and immune response. These habits not only foster menstrual health but also decrease cellular inflammation throughout your entire body. Taking care of your menstrual health before perimenopause and menopause will help you become healthier overall to navigate these life stages with more vitality and fewer symptoms.

Along with implementing nutritional and exercise recommendations, promote balance in your life by looking inward and understanding how you can honor your body and yourself throughout your entire menstrual cycle. Intend that your menstruation, the foods you eat, your rich inner life, your relationships, your work, and all your activities support you and bring you joy. Many Native Americans believe that women purify the earth through menstruation. See if connecting to your contribution to the planet by being a woman can help you deepen your power and appreciate yourself for all you do.

CHAPTER SEVEN

Endometriosis

Endometriosis, a non–life-threatening but debilitating condition that afflicts more than five million women in North America, occurs when the tissue that makes up the uterine lining—the endometrium—grows outside of the uterus. Throughout the reproductive years, the uterine lining cyclically grows to create a rich home for the fetus and then decomposes and is shed during menstruation if pregnancy does not occur. Endometriosis tissue also builds up and then breaks down during each menstrual cycle, similar to normal uterine lining. But because these cells are not in the uterus, the decaying material cannot be released from the body. Instead, the blood and other matter remain in the body, frequently forming cysts, nodules, adhesions, and scars on the organs, ligaments, and walls of the pelvic cavity.

The disease affects between 15 to 20 percent of American women of reproductive age. Risk factors include family history, short menstrual cycles, exposure to excess estrogen or estrogen disruptors, lack of exercise, a diet high in unhealthy fats, and possibly elevated stress levels. Women who have endometriosis may experience pain, menstrual problems, and infertility. Many women with the condition have chronic pelvic, abdominal, or lower back pain and experience pain with urination, bowel movements, sex, and digestion. Menstrual cramps that get

> Most women do experience a reduction of endometriosis symptoms at menopause, as long as they don't take HRT.

increasingly worse and become debilitating, along with heavy periods, spotting, and bleeding between periods, are also common.

Endometriosis is most frequently found in the pelvic cavity surrounding and attached to the uterus, bowels, ovaries, bladder, uterine ligaments, and pelvic walls. Endometriosis tissue may be referred to as lesions, implants, or nodules. In rare cases, endometriosis is found outside of the pelvis in the lungs and head. One doctor told me that he had a patient with endometriosis in her nose who would experience nosebleeds with each menstrual cycle.

Symptoms of endometriosis do not develop in any one standard manner and are not directly linked with the amount of endometriosis a woman has. Many women do not even realize they have endometriosis until they have difficulty becoming pregnant. Endometriosis diagnoses can take up to ten years because the condition presents symptoms similar to other conditions—particularly irritable bowel syndrome. Women with endometriosis are more likely to have chronic fatigue syndrome, autoimmune disorders, allergies, asthma, fibromyalgia, and hypothyroidism. Endometriosis does not cause cancer. However, in rare cases, women who have endometriosis can develop endometrioid cancer, so it is important to bring all endometriosis symptoms to the attention of your health care provider.

Infertility affects up to 40 percent of all women with endometriosis. Women who want to become pregnant are precluded from beginning or continuing many of the biomedical treatment options, as these would significantly lower their chances of successfully carrying a pregnancy to term.

Use the mind-body therapies in this chapter along with any biomedical techniques you choose to restore your hormonal balance, digestive tract, and immune system in order to reduce endometriosis symptoms and enhance fertility.

Biomedical Approaches to Endometriosis

Medical researchers do not know precisely what causes endometriosis. Different theories consider endometriosis an autoimmune disorder, a genetic problem, an endocrine disease, or a condition that results from retrograde menstrual flow, when tissue that is shed by the uterus with each period flows back into a woman's pelvis. Standard biomedical treatments include pain medication, hormone therapy, and surgical procedures.

Before establishing a treatment regimen, your physician will need to confirm your diagnosis. She or he will probably begin with a manual pelvic exam to feel for signs of endometriosis. Blood tests, an ultrasound, or an MRI generally follow this physical exam. All of these techniques can detect some endometriosis, but they also have limitations.

A definitive diagnosis for endometriosis can be obtained only through surgery. The most common procedure is a laparoscopy, in which the doctor makes a small incision in the abdomen and inserts the laparoscope, a small lighted instrument with a camera, to look inside the pelvis for endometriosis. The surgeon then biopsies a tissue sample to determine whether endometriosis is present. Some physicians prefer to treat pelvic pain for six months to see whether symptoms reduce without having to perform laparoscopy.

Your doctor may initially suggest pain medication as a first course of treatment. If your symptoms are mild, you will probably be advised to use over-the-counter or prescription nonsteroidal anti-inflammatory drugs (NSAIDs) such as ibuprofen or naproxen to manage pain. Even over-the-counter pain medication can have severe long-term side effects. If you do use pain relievers, consider doing so for just a few months while you implement new nutritional and lifestyle strategies to reduce pain and inflammation naturally, without the risks of detrimental side effects.

Estrogen accelerates endometriosis growth, so many hormonal treatments for the condition involve lowering estrogen levels. Your physician may recommend using hormonal contraceptives with estrogen or progestin to stop ovulation and reduce or cease menstruation. Gonadotropin-releasing hormone (GnRH) agonists are synthetic hormones that are frequently used to relieve endometriosis symptoms by artificially inducing menopause. GnRH medications such as Lupron or Synarel generally inhibit or diminish endometriosis growth within three months. GnRH medications can be used for only six months because of associated health risks and are generally followed by a course of hormonal contraceptives. Endometriosis recurrence is common after hormonal treatments are discontinued.

Treatment regimens that suppress ovulation may not be practical if you would like to conceive in the near future. GnRH drugs are expensive and have serious risks and side effects. Even if you have advanced endometriosis, you may obtain longer-term relief for a similar financial investment by working with an acupuncturist or massage or physical therapist with expertise relieving endometriosis in combination with implementing the holistic strategies outlined later in this chapter.

If you have severe endometriosis pain that has been unresponsive to medication, your physician may recommend surgery. Surgical options include laparoscopy and laparotomy with or without hysterectomy. Laparoscopic surgery for endometriosis involves several small incisions in the abdomen through which a surgeon uses the laparoscope to view the lesions and the interior of the pelvic cavity. The surgeon then either removes or destroys the endometriosis, while the surrounding tissue remains healthy and intact. This surgery is generally done on an outpatient basis, with a fairly quick recovery time. Laparotomy is considered major surgery that requires a hospital stay and six weeks to two months of recovery time. With a laparotomy, the surgeon makes a larger incision in the abdomen and may remove just the endometriosis tissue or the uterus, fallopian tubes, and ovaries as well.

Some women do get relief from endometriosis with surgery; others do not have positive results, even after multiple surgeries. Endometriosis recurrence is common with all types of surgery, even in the case of hysterectomy and ovarian removal, because endometriosis cells may be left in the body. If you are in extreme pain and feel that surgery is your best option, consider having laparoscopic surgery with a skilled physician to minimize the endometriosis tissue and scars in your body; then use holistic strategies to prevent recurrence by strengthening your immune and endocrine systems and decreasing your estrogen levels naturally. This may be an effective strategy for women who want to become pregnant. To improve fertility hindered by endometriosis, use the mind-body techniques in this chapter and chapter nine to nourish and restore your body.

Talking with Your Doctor

If you suspect you have endometriosis, find a doctor who will use diagnostic tools to determine the extent of your condition. Look for a gynecologist who understands the complex impact of endometriosis on women's lives.

Disclose all symptoms, including painful intercourse, bowel movements, and urination to your health care provider to help develop the best treatment regimen. If you are considering laparoscopic surgery, research physicians in your area to find someone skilled at pelviscopic techniques who has extensive experience removing or destroying endometriosis tissue.

Try not to be discouraged or internalize attitudes from physicians who may view endometriosis as untreatable or manageable only through hysterectomy or hormonal treatments that create early menopause. Keep on until you find the right caregiver for you. Many women find substantial relief from endometriosis pain and symptoms and restore

Choose a physician who works in partnership with pain specialists, nutritionists, counselors, and mind-body practitioners or, if you are interested in becoming pregnant, also specializes in endocrinology or infertility.

fertility though mind-body methods alone or in combination with medication or laparoscopy.

Holistic Approaches to Endometriosis

Holistic treatments for endometriosis focus on balancing the endocrine system, lowering dietary estrogens, detoxifying the body, reducing stress, and increasing vital energy. Biomedical organizations in Europe and some physicians in the United States are beginning to recognize the importance of using integrative treatments that address the emotional and physical stressors associated with endometriosis. In many cases, women with endometriosis feel out of control of their bodies and basic bodily processes. Endometriosis sufferers commonly become disillusioned and disappointed about the lack of effective medical treatments available. In a study of four thousand European women with endometriosis, researchers concluded that holistic treatments such as cognitive restructuring, counseling, nutrition, physical therapy, yoga, Pilates, and other hands-on manual therapies (such as massage) are frequently necessary to achieve long-term healing and quality of life.[1]

Endometriosis is a strong signal for women to take the time to nourish themselves. Mind-body approaches will not necessarily eliminate all endometriosis tissue, but they can provide significant symptom relief. Use the following modalities to diminish your symptoms, increase your energy, and improve your life. If you want to enhance your fertility, combine the information here with the strategies in chapter nine.

Nutrition, Supplements, and Herbs

Elizabeth was a thirty-two-year-old woman who came to see me about endometriosis and elevated stress in her life. She was reluctant to use the medication that her doctor suggested for her endometriosis because it would put her into early menopause. Along with stress-reduction tools, Elizabeth and I discussed the potential benefits of eliminating dairy, wheat, and meat from her diet while eating wild cold-water fish once or twice a week and increasing plant sources of protein for a few months to see whether these approaches might help with her pain.

After the first month, Elizabeth noticed that her symptoms were better than usual. By her third menstrual cycle on this diet, Elizabeth felt that the dietary changes combined with more exercise had significantly reduced her pain while increasing her energy. During the next month, Elizabeth experimented with adding dairy, wheat, and meat back into her diet. She found that she could eat hormone-free meat without reinitiating the pain, but when she started to eat wheat and dairy again, her symptoms flared up each time. Elizabeth loved yogurt, pizza, and pasta with cheese, but decided that avoiding the side effects of prescription medication was worth making these dietary changes permanently. When she had a longing for one of her old favorites, she found she could be satisfied with homemade cheese-free pizza with a brown rice flour crust, or a soy yogurt.

Like Elizabeth, many women with endometriosis find that making significant changes in their diet can eliminate pain. These changes can seem radical, as they often involve eating very differently than we are used to in the West. However, I encourage you to try these nutritional strategies in combination with the general recommendations in chapter four to heal and prevent endometriosis naturally.

When I was in Asia, I learned that the Chinese have a word for Europeans and Americans that translates into "people who smell like milk." Even though it may seem natural to us, many non-Western cultures have traditionally consumed very little dairy or meat. Regular dairy consumption can aggravate endometriosis symptoms for many women, and high levels of animal protein may elevate the risks of endometriosis. Italian researchers found that women who ate large amounts of beef, ham, or other red meats had an 80- to 100-percent increased risk of developing endometriosis.[2] Wheat consumption also exacerbates endometriosis symptoms in many cases.

If you are experiencing painful symptoms, eliminate dairy, meat, and wheat for two to four weeks or longer to see whether changing your diet eases your pain; the chemicals and hormones in these foods may be what inflames endometriosis tissue. Reintroduce organic dairy, organic non–genetically modified wheat, and hormone-free meat back into your diet on different weeks and see whether your symptoms return. Eat mostly fresh foods and avoid smoked, aged, and dried meats, fish, and cheese, and fermented foods and beverages such as soy sauce and beer. Keep a food diary to help track which foods cause pain.

Nutrition can be a powerful preventative and healing tool for endometriosis. Increase green leafy vegetables such as kale and bok choy, fresh fruit (other than citrus), beans, and healthy whole grains to boost your dietary fiber and reduce blood estrogen levels. Lessen inflammation by getting plenty of beneficial fatty acids from evening primrose oil, walnuts, ground flaxseeds, and krill oil while minimizing unhealthy fats. Eliminate sugar, alcohol, caffeine, and cigarettes. Use probiotics and other digestive enzymes to heal yeast and bowel problems common with endometriosis and help reduce allergy and chemical sensitivity. Eat foods rich in B vitamins, zinc, and magnesium. Take a multivitamin and a multimineral with magnesium, calcium, and zinc daily.

Consider following a whole-foods detoxification diet to clear chemicals from your body, as discussed in chapter four. Follow the recommendations in chapter two to reduce your contact with common chemicals and all toxic estrogen disruptors. (It is notable that in one study, monkeys exposed to the common environmental toxin dioxin developed high rates of endometriosis.[3])

Your skin plays an important role in eliminating toxins from your body. Experiment with dry skin brushing to help open up your pores and clean the lymphatic system. You can purchase a natural vegetable skin brush at your local health food store or on the Internet. Brush your dry skin each morning before a shower or bath with smooth, gentle, one-stroke movements, working from your hands and feet to the center of your body, covering the entire body below the neck just once. Use a softer dry skin brush for your face and gently brush from the center of your face outward and down the sides of your neck.

Herbal supplements to alleviate endometriosis symptoms include chaste tree, black cohosh, wild yam, crampbark, and dandelion. Chaste tree diminishes cramping, but it should not be combined with oral contraceptives, as it can lower their efficacy. Black cohosh can successfully lessen menstrual pain and inflammation, but do not use black cohosh during pregnancy, because it can cause miscarriage. Wild yam and crampbark decrease cramping and relax pelvic muscles. Dandelion supports liver function to detoxify the body.

Movement and Bodywork

In Chinese medicine traditions, endometriosis is frequently diagnosed as a condition of stagnant blood and energy or deficient energy. All types of enjoyable activities that get you moving and increase your energy will be beneficial. Exercise boosts endorphins (your body's natural pain relievers), decreases stress, and can lower estrogen levels. Movements that help improve pelvic circulation are an important component in restoring health and harmony for women with endometriosis. Yoga and Pilates include postural exercises that assist in opening up abdominal and pelvic areas for better blood flow and nervous system support while strengthening core muscles.

Swimming, walking, and restorative yoga are helpful exercises that you can do even if you are experiencing pain. Qi gong and tai chi can significantly reduce pain while providing you with better energy flow in your pelvic core. Squatting and bending during gardening or other activities can release stagnant pelvic energy and build flexibility. Stay away from jarring activities to prevent damage to endometrial scar tissue and lesions.

Stretching twice a day for ten to fifteen minutes will help relax sore muscles and rejuvenate energy. The Myofascial Energetic Length Technique (MELT) Method is an exercise program that uses foam rollers to heal and rehydrate abdominal and pelvic connective tissues affected by endometriosis adhesions. See the Resources section on page 221 for information about the MELT Method. Kegel exercises, described in chapter five, strengthen the internal pelvic muscles and reduce endometriosis pain for some women.

You may also want to seek assistance from a professional massage or physical therapist to help release endometriosis adhesions, ease pain, and free up pelvic energy. Working with massage therapists, acupuncturists, and other bodyworkers and energy healers has helped many women with endometriosis achieve pain relief and reverse infertility problems. Women who have pain during sex may want to have a physical evaluation to determine whether a tipped uterus is contributing to their problems. If so, treatments from a chiropractor or skilled bodyworker can help realign the uterus, frequently making intercourse more pleasurable.

Conscious Breathing

Use the instructions for abdominal breathing in chapter three to prepare for this deep breathing exercise. Relax, close your eyes, and focus your awareness on your endometriosis tissue. Breathe energy directly into all the areas of your body where your endometriosis exists. Imagine that you can sense the essence of the endometriosis cells. Notice any qualities about the endometriosis that emerge while you breathe, such as weight, sound, color, or texture. Ask the endometriosis whether it has any messages for you as you breathe in and out of it.

With every inhale, breathe healing light or energy to the endometriosis. Observe the cells becoming lighter and less dense. Let your exhales begin to slough the endometriosis away from your organs, ligaments, and connective tissue, and out of your body. Imagine that every breath loosens more and more of the endometriosis tissue and releases all pain. Continue to breathe deeply and feel your pelvis becoming lighter and freer. Continue this breathing practice for at least twenty minutes daily for three months, always with the intention that your endometriosis will detach and be released from your body. (Use the Second Chakra Breathing Exercise on page 129 to help strengthen your pelvic core.)

You can also use conscious breathing to bring more pleasure into your life. If you experience pain during intercourse because of your endometriosis, employ deep breathing during sexual play with yourself or a partner to see whether it can help you enjoy intimacy more fully. Consciously inhale pleasure, love, and light into your entire body while you exhale pain, tension, and fear from your pelvic cavity. Breathe deeply and fully as you explore different kinds of erotic pleasure that do not involve intercourse, to help your body relax and safely open back up to sex. When you are ready, try alternative positions, such as being on your hands and knees with your partner behind you, to take pressure off of areas that typically have higher concentrations of endometriosis tissue, or on top, where you can better control the depth and pace of penetration.

If you experience difficulties progressing with your conscious breathing practice, you may want to improve your indoor air quality. People with endometriosis often have increased sensitivity to airborne irritants, so eliminating these toxins is especially important. Reduce your exposure to mold, smoke, dust mites, and regular household cleaning and beauty products and consider using an effective air filter.

Cognitive Restructuring

We sometimes hold unconscious contracts about our bodies and/or lives that limit our pleasure, enjoyment, or ability to heal or achieve our dreams. This journaling exercise will help you become aware of any unconscious contracts you may have that restrict your joy or vitality. Take a few moments to consider whether you have any nonnourishing contracts about your health, body, relationships, career, or any other part of your life. Journal on what it would be like to establish new contracts that help you become your healthiest, happiest, and most successful self.

To help you formulate your new contracts, think about the qualities you would like to have in all the different areas of your life. This might be a commitment to support yourself with plenty of relaxing and rejuvenating activities that could help you heal. It might entail the choice to end, change, or limit your exposure to toxic relationships or career choices that compromise your health, and instead choosing to spend more time and energy on relationships and work that affirms your self-worth and beauty. You may simply want to surround yourself with more love, fun, ease, and richness. Journal about the energy and characteristics you would like to call into your life.

Make new contracts about your health, your body, your endometriosis recovery process, and your ability to heal and let go of pain. Writing down a contract or goal gives more energy to your intention. If you would like, copy your new contracts onto a piece of paper that you can keep and read them out loud to yourself every day for a month. If any part of a contract seems unattainable, use the "Four Steps to Change" process in chapter three to release any beliefs you may hold that are preventing you from easily fulfilling your contract.

Just as limiting exposure to toxic chemicals is vitally important for anyone with endometriosis, it is equally essential to detoxify your mind. To do this, focus your thoughts and language on love and gentleness for yourself and others. Shift your self-talk from a harsh or punishing dialogue to a compassionate conversation, with as many loving messages as possible. Fully feel any anger and regret about past situations and journal on ways to shift these patterns and the beliefs that contributed to them so you can open to receiving as much love as possible in the current moment. Release negative thinking habits, such as always assuming the worst, all-or-nothing thinking, and expecting a bleak future.

In my work with clients, I have seen how living with chronic pain such as endometriosis can result in a tendency to focus on the fear of the future rather than thinking about all the good things your future holds. If you regularly think about your health getting worse and how this will affect your life and your ability to achieve your goals and dreams, write a new contract for your future and use this exercise to help build a strong relationship with your most joyous future. When you concentrate on the fear of the future, you are actually giving more energy to the future you do not want.

To help shift this energy, begin to focus on finding the solutions to your problems in the future. Start to observe how you think about the future throughout your day. When you find yourself focusing on a mediocre or dark future, connect to the feelings and beliefs that are creating this future outcome. Journal on the different ways you relate to the future. Write about why you choose to view your future the way you do and how you will feel if you choose to focus your awareness on your future taking shape in a way that fully supports you and your deepest goals and desires.

Visualization

In *Guided Imagery for Self-Healing*, physician Martin Rossman describes how a woman healed herself of endometriosis by visualizing her lesions as tar attached to her abdominal organs.[4] For three months, she took fifteen minutes two or three times a day to envision cleaning up all of the tar using a scraper, cleaning solution, and a mop. When her gynecologist examined her pelvic cavity with laparoscopy afterward, she had no visible traces of endometriosis.

Healing Endometriosis Visualization: Following the general guidelines for guided imagery in chapter three, employ visualizations like the one described above to imagine your endometriosis releasing from your body. You may want to envision a gentle vacuum programmed only to take in unhealthy cells that sucks up and removes your endometriosis from your entire body. Or you could feel cleansing water flowing through your pelvic cavity, breaking up and releasing your implants from your organs and other tissue. Breathe deeply and picture your body being free of all endometriosis. Imagine what it feels like to be totally healed. Know that your uterus is in perfect balance. Envisage your endometrial lining being in harmony with the rest of your body, existing only inside your uterus.

Choose whatever imagery feels best to you and use it consistently at least twice a day for twenty minutes, for three months or longer. Near the end of each imagery session, take a few moments to sense that your body, immune system, and liver are already strong and healthy. Feel yourself receiving nourishment and releasing nonnourishing energy, as well as restoring overall vitality. Use this visualization to accompany any surgical procedure or pharmaceutical treatment you undergo for endometriosis. Imagine the technology permanently eliminating all implants and adhesions in a safe and effective way.

You can also use imagery to help minimize the pain associated with endometriosis. Begin by connecting with the pain using your curiosity. Ask yourself how the pain would look if it were an image. What kind of action does the pain feel like it is doing to you? You might imagine that the pain is a hand, an adhesive substance, or a metal instrument that is constricting or squeezing your body or your internal organs, or you might see or feel that it is something or someone hitting, kicking, poking, prodding, or hurting you in some other manner.

Trust your senses and go with the feelings or images that come to you, or use one of the descriptions in the preceding paragraph to relate to your pain. Once you have an impression of the pain, ask the pain what it is trying to tell you or communicate to you. As you breathe deeply in your visualization, really observe or listen to the pain as if it has something important to tell you.

Ask your pain any questions that arise into your consciousness. Imagine that you are finally able to have an important conversation or communication with a sacred part of yourself that has vital information that can help you restore yourself back to health. Fully feel everything you have felt about your pain and openly tell your pain anything you want to say to it. Ask the pain whether there are any beliefs that you can release to facilitate and quicken your healing process. Even if you do not get any clear information during the visualizations, know that taking the time to communicate with your body in a nonjudgmental manner will help you access your inner wisdom and healing insights during your recovery.

After you have taken the time to allow your body to communicate with you, use your imagination to reverse the image or action that is hurting you. If you see your pain as someone or something such as a metal vise squeezing your organs, envision this object or grip letting go. Let your entire abdomen and pelvis relax and feel good. Release the constriction, the pain, and the object causing the discomfort from your consciousness and body. If you envisioned your own hands or a disempowered part of you causing the pain or holding the pain-producing object, envision your hands or this part of yourself rejuvenated and fulfilled, engaged in a beneficial activity such as painting, meditation, or any fun or creative pursuit you enjoy. If you pictured someone other than yourself creating the pain, imagine them releasing from your being completely. Feel the release fully.

As you do this, imagine that you can reclaim any personal power and vital energy that you gave to your pain and to whatever or whoever you symbolically visualized causing it. See any energy or power that you surrendered to your pain returning to or remaining in your body, purified by the golden light of intention, while all the pain and the energy, beliefs, and feelings connected to it leave your consciousness, body, and home.

Sense soothing, beautiful energy flowing into your body, filling up the area from which you released the painful energy. Allow yourself to breathe deeply into the comfort and space that has opened up inside your body. Many women experience an immediate decrease in pain when they do this visualization. To reduce your pain as much as possible, continue the visualization twice a day for fifteen to twenty minutes for three months.

A Brighter Future

A growing body of evidence supports the effectiveness of holistic health techniques in reducing endometriosis pain and inflammation on its own or as a complement to biomedical treatments. The successes of nutritional healing and manipulative therapies such as physical therapy and massage provide new directions for women with endometriosis to use in combination with standard treatments or when side effects are undesirable or treatment options would significantly lower the chances of successfully carrying a pregnancy to term. Honor yourself by bringing these healing techniques into your life. They will help you decrease endometriosis symptoms, improve fertility, and more fully enjoy your body.

CHAPTER EIGHT

Fibroids

Uterine fibroids are noncancerous tumors that affect millions of women. The majority of fibroids produce no problematic symptoms, yet these benign tumors are the number one reason for hysterectomy in the United States. Each year more than three hundred thousand U.S. women have hysterectomies on account of fibroids, even though studies show that uterine removal is medically unnecessary in most cases. There are an increasing number of less-invasive medical treatments and complementary therapies that women can use to either remove fibroids or decrease symptoms, allowing them to keep their uteruses.

Thirty percent of all American women ages twenty-five to forty-five are diagnosed with uterine fibroids, and it is estimated that more than 70 percent of all reproductive-age women in the United States have fibroids, many of them undiagnosed. Increased risk factors include family history, excessive stress, diets high in refined foods, early age of menarche, not having children, and obesity. African-American women are three to nine times more likely to develop uterine fibroids than women of other ethnicities.

Uterine fibroids range in size from a quarter inch to six or more inches in diameter. When medical practitioners describe fibroid dimensions, they generally compare the size of the uterus and fibroids together to either a representative fruit (orange, grapefruit, even cantaloupe in severe cases) or fetal development ("the size of a five-month-old fetus"). Fibroid growth accelerates during pregnancy, when hormonal levels are high. Uterine fibroids usually get smaller and less symptomatic as women go through menopause and levels of estrogen decline, as long as no estrogen therapy is used.

Most women may not realize they have uterine fibroids until told by a doctor during an exam. Yet others experience debilitating pain, bleeding, and bloating before their diagnosis. Many fibroid sufferers in my study reported having severely heavy menstrual periods, pelvic pain, anemia, urinary problems, pain during sex, and pressure in the uterus and surrounding organs. In some cases, uterine fibroids can result in infertility or problems during pregnancy, including miscarriage. Although, again, fibroid tumors are noncancerous, they can present symptoms similar to those of cancer, such as abnormal bleeding, abdominal bloating, and bleeding between periods, which is one reason some doctors choose to remove the uterus once fibroids are detected.

Biomedical Approaches to Uterine Fibroids

Medical researchers know relatively little about why uterine fibroids develop. The extent of symptoms and pain experienced generally corresponds to tumor location and size. Fibroids found underneath the uterine lining or embedded in the uterine wall will frequently produce heavy menstrual bleeding. Fibroids that degenerate because they get cut off from the blood supply or for other reasons will cause pain. Large fibroid tumors that block fertilized egg implantation or impede fetal growth can increase risk for infertility and miscarriage in some cases. Fibroids are generally considered estrogen dependent, so excess estrogen can speed fibroid growth.

Before you take any steps to treat fibroids, first be sure to get screened for cervical, endometrial, and ovarian cancer.

There are a variety of biomedical treatments for fibroids. Your choice of treatment—whether by using solely holistic methods or in combination with Western medical technologies—will probably depend on the intensity of your symptoms and your personal philosophy. Some women with fibroids experience bleeding so heavy that for several days each month they cannot leave the house even to go to work. In cases such as these, severe pain or dangerously low blood iron levels can make the woman too exhausted to implement the lifestyle changes needed to reduce symptoms though mind-body techniques.

If you face similar challenges, you may want to use biomedical treatments that will rapidly moderate any dangerous symptoms; then, as you regain your strength, you can begin to integrate whole-foods nutrition, stress reduction, and exercise into your life. Consider first trying approaches that have the lowest risks and can be easily reversed, to see whether they provide you with relief before choosing more invasive, higher-risk options.

Watchful waiting can be used for fibroids that are not creating pain, excessive bleeding, or other complications. Asymptomatic fibroids can simply be monitored annually with a pelvic exam and do not require treatment. If you can easily tolerate your fibroids, use the mind-body strategies in this book to help prevent problematic symptoms from developing.

Nonsteroidal anti-inflammatory drugs (NSAIDs) such as ibuprofen are frequently recommended to alleviate fibroid pain and moderate heavy bleeding. Some physicians prescribe stronger NSAIDs and may combine these pain-relieving drugs with hormonal contraceptives to further reduce fibroid symptoms. However, regular use of over-the-counter

If you are near menopause and not in distress from fibroids, you can wait before undergoing any invasive procedure to see whether lower estrogen levels help shrink fibroids naturally to provide you with relief.

and prescription NSAIDs can cause serious intestinal and kidney damage. NSAIDs reduce pain by blocking inflammatory prostaglandin production in the uterus. To get the same anti-inflammatory and menstrual regulating results through a safer long-term method, adopt the nutrition strategies and the mind-body healing techniques presented here and limit any NSAIDs to short-term use.

Estrogen and progestin are often prescribed to regulate abnormal bleeding caused by fibroids, but both of these treatments have potential side effects. Progestin reduces heavy bleeding by encouraging frequent shedding of the uterine lining, but it may induce fibroid growth. Some biomedical authorities believe that estrogen causes fibroids and recommend that women with fibroids should not use estrogen to control bleeding, for contraceptives, or for menopausal symptoms. However, physicians commonly prescribe oral contraceptives containing estrogen to lessen bleeding and reduce pain from fibroids. Progestin contraceptives such as Depo-Provera and progestin-reducing IUDs are also used to decrease heavy bleeding caused by fibroids. Because estrogen and progestin may both contribute to fibroid development, request an ultrasound before embarking on any hormonal treatment, and have another a few months after starting estrogen or progestin to monitor the status of your fibroids.

GnRH analogs are synthetic hormones that shrink fibroids by inhibiting pituitary function to stop ovarian estrogen production and induce sudden, reversible menopause. Lupron, Zoladex, and Synarel are GnRH analog drugs that can be used for up to six months to stop bleeding to stabilize blood iron count, and to minimize fibroids so that they are small enough to be removed without hysterectomy. Once GnRH drugs are stopped, fibroid reccurrence accelerates quickly. This treatment can be very expensive and may pose serious risks even when used for just a few months.

Currently, hysterectomy is still the most frequent biomedical treatment for fibroids, but the past decade has seen an increase of less-invasive surgical procedures. There is a complete discussion of hysterectomy in chapter eleven; all of the other procedures for removing or shrinking fibroids in this chapter leave the uterus in the body.

Myomectomy—the surgical removal of fibroids that can be performed through traditional surgery, hysteroscopy, or laparoscopy—is the safest surgical fibroid treatment available for women who still want to have children. Uterine fibroid embolization, commonly called UFE, shrinks fibroid tumors through the injection of tiny plastic or gelatin-based particles into the artery supplying blood to the fibroid. UFE is performed by a radiologist and has a low rate of fibroid recurrence. In an outpatient procedure using a device called the ExAblate, radiologists can use MRI-guided focused ultrasound surgery (FUS) to direct high-frequency ultrasound waves at the uterus to break up fibroids. FUS just takes a few hours, and recovery typically takes just a few days. For the majority of women treated, fibroid symptoms usually decrease within a few months, but can return over time.

Myomectomy, UFE, and FUS offer women alternative ways to remove fibroids to provide substantial relief while still retaining the uterus. However, each of these options come with potential side effects including pelvic pain, loss of blood supply to the uterus, infertility, infection, and early onset of menopause. If you are interested in becoming pregnant in the future, do not use UFE or FUS; the long-term effects of these procedures on fertility and the uterus are currently unknown. Even though each of these procedures poses some risks to uterine health, they will allow you to keep your uterus and benefit from its many functions.

Talking with Your Doctor

Consult your doctor at the onset of any problems with fibroids, such as heavy bleeding and pain, so you can try the least-invasive medical treatment possible and use complementary options before your condition becomes too serious. Bring a record of the intensity and frequency of your symptoms to all health care appointments to help you and your doctor assess which treatment options are best for you.

If your symptoms are not debilitating, inform your doctor that you would like to employ watchful waiting, explore pharmaceutical treatments to control symptoms, or undergo less-invasive surgical options first to remove fibroids without having to remove the uterus. If your doctor presents hysterectomy as the only option for treating fibroids, seek a second opinion or a different physician.

If you are deciding between a hysterectomy or a less-invasive procedure to remove your uterine fibroids, become fully informed about the best surgeons and radiologists available in your area who frequently perform these procedures. Make a list of all the reasons in favor of and against each treatment option. If you would like to reduce your symptoms without the risks or side effects of medications or invasive procedures, give yourself a few months to integrate holistic approaches into your life. If you do choose to have your fibroids surgically removed or have a hysterectomy, use the exercise, nutritional, and stress-reduction strategies in this book to help prevent fibroid regrowth or make hysterectomy recovery as easy as possible.

Holistic Approaches for Uterine Fibroids

Holistic treatments for fibroids focus on balancing the endocrine system, clearing stagnant pelvic energy, and decreasing dietary estrogen. From a mind-body perspective, excessive estrogen levels caused by the typical Western lifestyle contribute to our high rates of uterine fibroids. Integrative approaches in this chapter and in the Optimal Uterine Health Plan (part two) will help you alleviate fibroid symptoms by balancing your estrogen levels and lowering stress.

Complementary techniques can reduce fibroid symptoms and size and prevent new fibroids from developing, but they will not usually make fibroids go away. If you have difficult symptoms from fibroids and you wish to use only natural treatments for your condition, you may want to seek the assistance of an acupuncturist, homeopath, breath coach, massage therapist, or energy healer in addition to pursuing the self-help practices presented here to accelerate your healing process.

Nutrition, Supplements, and Herbs

Most fibroids are thought to feed on estrogen. Diets high in refined foods, saturated and trans fats, and conventional meat and dairy create excess estrogen conditions in the body. Alcohol consumption, B vitamin deficiency, red meat, and obesity are risk factors for fibroids. Implement the nutritional recommendations outlined in chapter four to increase fiber, lower your dietary estrogen levels, boost your nutrient intake, and prevent weight gain. To help reduce pain and excessive bleeding from fibroids, you will want to follow these dietary guidelines as closely as possible for at least three to six months.

Eat mostly organic vegetables, fruit, beans, and whole grains, and eliminate as much refined food, sugars, dairy, unhealthy oils, alcohol, and caffeine as you can. Increase your beneficial fats by eating omega-3-rich foods such as ground flaxseed, walnuts, and wild cold-water fish. Omega-3 fatty acids decrease tumors in animals, and dietary flaxseed has been shown to shrink tumor growth in women with breast cancer.[1] Eat plenty of these beneficial fats daily for three months to see whether your fibroid symptoms can be eased with increased omega-3 levels.

Cook with plenty of medicinal herbs, such as turmeric, ginger, and garlic, to enhance your immune system. Once you notice an improvement with fibroid pain and bleeding, you can see whether starting to eat organic dairy products again produces pain for you. If not, add organic dairy back into your diet in moderation, if you wish. Discontinuing dairy altogether for a few months will help lower your estrogen levels and give your uterus a chance to heal.

Lycopene, the pigment that gives tomatoes and some other fruits their red color, has antioxidant properties that may help reduce the size and incidence of fibroids. Research shows that lycopene supplementation in

Holistic approaches can take longer than conventional medical treatments, so give mind-body techniques at least two to three months to begin to take effect.

animals for more than nine months shrinks fibroids and lessens their occurrence.[2] Studies with humans are not complete yet, but you can see whether you benefit from increased lycopene in your diet by eating a variety of watermelon, papaya, pink grapefruit, and cooked tomatoes daily. Raw tomatoes combined with a healthy fat, such as extra-virgin olive oil, and fresh-squeezed tomato juice also provide ample lycopene. If you have your fibroids removed through myomectomy or another procedure, eat plenty of lycopene-rich foods while implementing a low-estrogen diet, herbal support, stress reduction, and regular exercise to prevent recurrence.

Supplement with cold-pressed borage oil or evening primrose oil to obtain beneficial omega-6 fatty acids. Women with excessive bleeding will want to eat plenty of iron-rich foods, such as blackstrap molasses, leafy greens, and sea vegetables, or take an iron supplement to prevent anemia. Take a multivitamin, magnesium, and an additional B vitamin complex. Use inositol and choline supplements to support the liver in removing fat from the body and lowering estrogen levels.

Herbs can help slow fibroid growth and minimize their size. It may be several months to a year before you will see results from herbal remedies, but generally fibroids grow rather slowly, so if you are not having serious problems, herbs might be effective for you. If you have asymptomatic fibroids, herbs can be a great way to avert future fibroid problems. A variety of herbs can improve fibroid symptoms. Chaste tree and skullcap taken daily for at least nine months can help reduce fibroid size. Red raspberry rejuvenates the uterus and can decrease bleeding. Use milk thistle, burdock root, and dandelion as herbal tinctures or daily teas to strengthen your liver and improve estrogen metabolization, digestion, and elimination. Stay away from dong quai (unless advised to take it by your health care provider), as it can increase blood flow during menstruation.

In addition to making dietary changes, limit your estrogen and synthetic progestin exposure as much as possible. Do not use long-term hormonal contraceptives, avoid menopausal hormone therapy, and limit contact with estrogen-disrupting chemicals as discussed in chapter two. Dr. Christiane Northrup recommends using natural or bioidentical progesterone for women who cannot make nutritional changes as well as those whose fibroid symptoms remain after implementing a whole-foods diet.[3] Northrup states that natural progesterone provides the same benefits as the synthetic hormone without as many side effects, such as headaches and bloating for most women. However, others believe that even natural progesterone can increase fibroid size.

Movement and Bodywork

Regular exercise can help prevent fibroids from developing in the first place. Walking, running, swimming, yoga, Pilates, and weight training are ideal exercises for women who are not experiencing major health issues from fibroids. Dance and other movement forms discussed in chapter five (such as Rosen Method Movement, Nia, and Feldenkrais) can provide a wonderful workout while also strengthening the mind-body connection. Exercise at least four times a week for thirty minutes to an hour. Discuss your exercise plan with your doctor if you have any health concerns.

Gentle yoga can help decrease pain from fibroids and open up the energy of the abdomen. Yogic poses such as twists, supported bridge pose, and forward bends can be particularly soothing for women with fibroids. Do not do inversions while menstruating, and avoid demanding yoga poses or styles that can strain your body during your healing process. Regular stretching for five to ten minutes twice a day will also help reduce pain and relax tight muscles and connective tissue.

If you choose to have surgery to remove fibroids, talk to your doctor to determine the right exercise program for you to follow to increase your stamina before your procedure. Moderate exercise before surgery can improve your recovery time. Give your body plenty of time to heal after surgery and always discuss your postoperative exercise plan with your physician before starting to work out. Walking and gentle mind-body exercises such as tai chi, qi gong, or restorative yoga can be safe ways to gradually resume exercising once your physician tells you it is safe to begin moderate forms of movement. Start gradually and refrain from weight lifting and abdominal exercises for several months.

Many women find relief from fibroid symptoms through acupressure, massage therapy, acupuncture, and other energy healing modalities. These treatments may not reduce the size of your fibroids, but they can help reduce pain, strengthen your immune and endocrine systems, and clear blocked energy. Find a healer who has experience helping women with uterine fibroids.

Conscious Breathing

High stress can lead to accelerated fibroid growth. The beauty of the breath is that you can use it to reduce stress wherever you are. One reason that conscious breathing has been used for thousands of years as the primary cornerstone of so many healing traditions is its portability. Anywhere you go, you can deepen your breath to help relax, rejuvenate, and restore your body.

Conscious breathing is very helpful to employ during or after interactions that leave you stressed out or depleted. When you find yourself under a great deal of stress, take a moment to reconnect with your breathing. On your inhale, breathe in peace and nourishment. With your exhale, let go of exhaustion, fear, and stress. If you like, visualize a place that helps you feel calm, such as a beautiful forest or the beach. Breathe like this for a few minutes and feel the relaxation in your body.

Along with being a wonderful stress-reduction tool, conscious breathing can assist you in connecting deeply with your body. You can use the uterine breathing exercise presented in chapter three to get in touch with the emotional energy in your fibroids. Start by following the uterine breathing process, which employs diaphragmatic breathing. As you breathe into your uterus, begin to focus your awareness on your fibroids. You can choose to concentrate on one fibroid or all of them—do what feels right for you. Imagine that you are actually breathing into your fibroids. Start to sense the energy within your fibroids. Know that you can become fully conscious of your fibroids—they are part of you; you are one.

As you breathe deeply into your fibroids, invite them to communicate whatever it is they would like to tell you. Ask them what they need. Believe that you can fully open up to your own inner guidance and understand why this condition developed. Stay open and compassionate. Ask your fibroids what will help them stop growing, causing pain, or creating abnormal bleeding and what you can do to help.

Continue to breathe deeply and allow yourself to fully feel any emotions or energy that are stored in your fibroids. Let yourself truthfully feel however you feel, even if it is anger, sadness, or disappointment at yourself or others or any emotion you may have repressed in the past. Breathe and feel the feelings that are emerging—knowing that being conscious to this energy will heal it.

Go ahead and also feel any anger or frustration you have felt toward your fibroids or yourself for the pain and discomfort they have caused. Be totally honest about your feelings. Inquire about the beliefs you hold that may have shaped your experience with fibroids. Know that you are powerful; you can change your beliefs and create a reality full of vitality, support, and compassion, and forgive yourself, your body, others, the world, and your fibroids. Breathe love and forgiveness to your fibroids, your uterus, and your entire being and breathe out any repressed emotions or energy from your fibroids and uterus. Ask your uterus what treatments or new understandings will help you establish total health. Breathe any insights or new empowered beliefs into your fibroids and uterus and throughout your whole body.

This may be a totally new way for you to relate to your body and fibroids. Give yourself several opportunities to open up to your inner wisdom by repeating this exercise weekly or more often for a few months. You may not initially experience any powerful shifts during your breathing, but insights about your health may eventually appear to you in other ways. If strong emotions arise during this process, you may be tempted to stop this conscious breathing exercise. Be assured that the breath is not creating your feelings—it is simply helping you become aware of the energy in your body. Continue your conscious breathing sessions regularly until you have released any repressed emotions from your fibroids and uterus and feel peaceful during the breathing process. Keep your journal nearby to write down any insights that come to you during each session, and journal for a few minutes after breathing, if you would like.

Cognitive Restructuring

Make some time in your life to examine your beliefs about fibroids and your ability to heal. One helpful way to do this is to journal about your fibroids. Write about what your fibroids mean to you, including how you feel about them and how your feelings have changed over time. Be completely honest. If you are angry at the world or yourself or someone else because you have to deal with fibroids, go ahead and write how you really feel. Let all of your emotions flow out of your body into your journal, knowing that you can come back and read it afterward.

Imagine that you are able to completely connect with your fibroids. Without thinking, write in a stream of consciousness anything your fibroids would like to communicate to you. You can ask your fibroids, uterus, or body to speak to you through your journaling. Let anything that comes up flow onto the page—even if it doesn't make logical sense to you. Draw an image or make a collage if words do not emerge. Make a collage or write about how you will feel and what you will do when you no longer experience bothersome symptoms from fibroids.

Some energy medicine practitioners believe that healing uterine fibroids can be facilitated by freely expressing creativity and emotions in life and relationships. You may find it helpful to use journaling to reveal any beliefs that have blocked you from easily expressing your creativity, wants, needs, and desires to yourself, your loved ones, and the world. While journaling, ask yourself what it would be like to let your creativity flow and to feel safe honestly expressing yourself in all your interactions. Journal on the messages you learned from your family when you were growing up about the proper ways for girls and women to communicate, behave, and relate to others. Let yourself write about new methods of self-expression, creativity, and interpersonal dynamics that more fully reflect the woman you have become.

Journal on what your life would look like if all your wants and desires came true. Connect with this on a feeling level and truthfully examine how you will feel when you create all of your dreams and desires. If you uncover any discomfort or insecurities about fulfilling your wants and desires, journal on the attitudes that might be creating these unsafe feelings. Write new beliefs that you would like to establish in your life.

You may also want to identify any feelings that are typically difficult for you to fully experience. This could be sadness, anger, or even enthusiasm or excitement. Use the "Four Steps to Change" in chapter three to reveal the beliefs that create challenges to authentic expression or any other difficulty you are currently experiencing.

Imagine what it would be like to be able to easily feel and express creative energy in your life. Allow yourself to feel all your emotions throughout your day. Recognize that you do not have to react to your feelings; instead, you can be present to them, becoming aware of how you feel in different situations and noticing what your beliefs are when you feel a certain way.

Visualization

Follow the general guidelines for visualization in chapter three. Always take a few moments to relax and breathe deeply in a peaceful place when you begin any guided imagery and continue breathing fully during your visualization. This visualization script will be most effective if you first do the exercises in the conscious breathing and cognitive restructuring sections of this chapter.

Visualization for Uterine Fibroids: You can use visualization to get in touch with the energy of your fibroids. Envision all the qualities of your fibroids. Ask yourself, if my fibroids had a color, what color would it be? If my fibroids made a noise, what sound would it be? If my fibroids had an odor, what would the smell be? If my fibroids had a taste, what flavor would it be? If my fibroids were an emotion, what emotion would it be? If my fibroids were a texture, what would the texture be? If my fibroids were an element (earth, air, fire, water), what element would they be? If my fibroids had a vibration, what would it be? If my fibroids could communicate to me, what would they want to tell me?

Deeply connect with any feelings, energy, messages, or meanings that emerge during this guided imagery. See whether you can communicate with your body and understand the patterns that caused the fibroids to develop (this might be genetics, exposure to chemicals, nutrition, stress, or something else) and steps you can take to heal. Honor your inner knowledge and express gratitude to your body.

Imagine what it would be like to release these energies and emotions from your uterus. Envision the various qualities that emerged about your fibroids (color, sound, texture, smell, and so on) and sense these energies leaving your body. Sense yourself releasing anger, hurt, guilt, rage, and all other unexpressed and buried emotions safely and healthfully while receiving creativity, inspiration, love, and support. Feel the energies letting go; help them, if need be, by imagining water or air flowing through and clearing these qualities from your uterus and life.

Next, begin to visualize your fibroids getting smaller and dissolving. If you have multiple fibroids, you may want to focus on one fibroid at a time shrinking and releasing from your uterus, or you may wish to imagine all your fibroids leaving at once. Do what feels right to you. Either way, envision your fibroids getting softer, smaller, and more permeable. You might like to envisage your fibroids melting or turning into liquid and leaving your body. You might picture your fibroids becoming dry, like chalk that turns to powder and begins to dissipate and flow out of your uterus, body, and home and into the earth. Or you can imagine your fibroids leaving in some other way. Perhaps you sense yourself safely cutting (or removing in another way) the fibroids from their base and easily releasing them from your uterus and body. You may also want to envision your uterus free of fibroids.

Susan was a thirty-seven-year-old woman with uterine fibroids that were causing her pain. She chose to address the condition through natural means, so she and her physician decided to take a watchful waiting approach, monitoring her fibroids regularly with an ultrasound. Before she came to see me, Susan had already implemented a whole-foods diet that helped stabilize her bleeding, but she still was in pain. Through conscious breathing and visualization sessions, Susan got in touch with the energy in her fibroids and realized that she had a lot of repressed anger in her uterus.

Our work helped Susan uncover her feelings and recognize the beliefs that were creating both the anger in her life and her fears about freely expressing herself. Susan came to realize that her open self-expression would actually create new growth and beauty in her life. Accordingly, she envisioned releasing her anger and the fibroids into the ground, where they would transform and nourish a lovely young tree. She used this visualization daily for many weeks and eventually turned it in to a ritual, actually planting a beautiful flowering tree in the place she had pictured in her imagery. Susan's pain gradually decreased until she no longer felt any discomfort or the bulge where her fibroids had been. At her next OB/GYN appointment, to her own surprise, the ultrasound revealed that her uterus was fibroid-free.

Visualization will not generally completely eliminate fibroids as it did for Susan, but if used consistently it can be a powerful tool for reducing fibroid pain and symptoms, especially when used alongside the nutritional, exercise, and stress-reduction recommendations in this chapter. Choose whatever imagery for dissolving and clearing fibroids feels best to you. Use it daily for at least twenty minutes for three months. If you focus on one fibroid at a time, be sure to continue your visualization process with all of your fibroids.

You can also use guided imagery to envision nutrition, herbs, medications, or surgical procedures working beautifully. Imagine that the foods you eat and any herbs, medications, or surgery shrink and release your fibroids. See your menstruation regulating and your uterus and pelvis feeling great. Picture yourself as totally healthy and happy in both the near and the distant future, imagining that your dietary and lifestyle changes and any medications or surgery will leave you well and full of energy.

Cultivating Freedom of Expression

Use the many holistic strategies in this book to prevent and relieve symptoms from uterine fibroids. Each of these techniques blends easily with biomedical treatments to strengthen your body and enhance your innate healing ability. Trust your inner wisdom to know which of these will work best for your own body.

In mind-body traditions, the uterus is viewed as the center of creative expression. The approaches in this chapter will enable you to tap into your own creative power to heal and transform your body. These modalities will also help you open up to enjoyable ways of expressing yourself in your interactions with others. Explore new means of self-expression, such as art, dance, and journaling. Celebrate the health you already enjoy and envision yourself strong and fit throughout your entire life.

CHAPTER NINE

Fertility, Pregnancy, and Birth

A healthy uterus is vitally important for successful conception, pregnancy, and birth. The uterus provides a home for the newly formed zygote and life support for the developing fetus, and it moves the baby out of the body in the birthing process. Our modern lifestyles create physiological challenges and high levels of stress that can make it more difficult to conceive or have a healthy pregnancy and an easy birth. Use the holistic strategies outlined in this chapter to support your endocrine system, balance hormones, and reduce stress, to facilitate each stage of this process.

Nearly 90 percent of all sexually active couples in the United States in their fertile years who do not use contraception will conceive within a year. However, more than 10 percent of all women have compromised fertility, and more than 20 percent of all pregnancies end in miscarriage. Even though it is not often recognized, more than one-quarter of all couples' fertility problems result from male infertility. Most impairments of female fertility stem from either tubal obstructions or difficulties with ovulation. Uterine problems, endometriosis, deteriorated egg supply, chromosomal dysfunction, compromised immune function, exposure to toxins, and other, unexplained causes can also affect female fertility.

The fallopian tubes transport eggs from the ovary to the uterus for conception and implantation. Pelvic infections, previous pelvic surgery, and endometriosis adhesions can cause tubal dysfunction, responsible for 40 percent of female infertility. Many tubal obstructions and ovulation problems can be healed by using the strategies in this book, in combination with treatments from a physical therapist, deep tissue massage therapist, acupuncturist, chiropractor, or energy healer.

The mind-body strategies presented here will help you navigate the terrain of pregnancy and birth with increased confidence. In the United States, pregnancy and birth have become highly medicalized. Cesarean section is the most common surgery in this country. According to the Centers for Disease Control press release of March 18, 2009, "The cesarean delivery rate rose 2 percent in 2007, to 31.8 percent, marking the eleventh consecutive year of increase and another record high for the United States." C-sections can be lifesavers for both mother and child in emergency cases; however, they are major surgeries, with significant risks and recovery time for the mother. Most births will progress safely on their own without medical intervention.

It is important to remember that throughout human history most women have had successful pregnancies and births without the assistance of our current technical advances—otherwise our species would not have been able to continue as it has. Trust that your body knows what to do: you just need to offer nourishment and energy to assist it. Pregnancy and birth are both based on healthy uterine functions. Use the tools in this chapter and the Optimal Uterine Health Plan (part two) to tone your uterus and create a healthy, joyful pregnancy and birth experience.

Biomedical Approaches to Fertility, Pregnancy, and Birth

Conventional medical methods to increase fertility include hormonal treatments, surgical procedures, and assisted reproductive technologies. If you do not conceive after a year of regular, unprotected sex, or six

Begin using nutrition and stress-reduction techniques for several months up to a year, if possible, before you want to conceive to improve uterine and endocrine function and enhance conception, pregnancy, and birth.

months if you're over thirty-five, biomedical practitioners will recommend diagnostic exams and hormone tests for you and your partner to determine what is obstructing fertility. Problems range from structural impairments such as scarring on the fallopian tubes that blocks transport of sperm and egg, to hormonal imbalances that compromise sperm and egg production and quality.

Medications that induce ovulation, such as Clomid, aromatase inhibitors, and gonadotropin, are frequently used either alone or to enhance intrauterine insemination (IUI). These medications often increase the chance of multiple gestations and have certain risks for the uterus or ovaries, so you may want to first employ whole-foods nutrition and mind-body tools to jump-start ovulation naturally. Laparoscopic surgery may be used with medications in cases of endometriosis to remove adhesions that impair fertility (see chapter seven for more on this procedure).

A variety of assisted reproductive technologies (ART) are used in combination with medications to increase conception when other techniques have not worked. During IUI, sperm is transferred into the uterus during ovulation. With in vitro fertilization (IVF), sperm and eggs are combined in a laboratory dish. After fertilization, the embryo is placed in the uterus. Intra-cytoplasmic insemination (ICSI), in which the sperm is injected into the egg, is frequently used with IVF. All of these ART processes are generally very stressful physically, emotionally, and financially for most people. Success is possible, but rates are low.

During pregnancy, your physician or midwife will see you for regular prenatal visits that become more frequent as the pregnancy progresses. Attending all of your prenatal check-ups is important in order to monitor your health and the health of your baby. If you are using a midwife, schedule at least one of your prenatal visits with the obstetrician who

Working with a mind-body healer can significantly improve the outcome of conventional fertility treatments.

will assist your midwife in the event that a physician is needed during the birth.

The biomedical approach to birth is based on a series of high-tech practices used to maintain the health of the baby and the mother. In emergencies, biomedicine provides a valuable service for mother and child. However, in this system the progress of birth is based on the hospital's schedule rather than the baby's schedule. Many of the medical procedures regularly used during birth—such as epidurals, encouraging women to remain in bed, and delivering with the woman flat on her back with her feet up in stirrups—actually impede labor and eventually cause more medical interventions to bring the baby into the world. The United States has the most technologically advanced approach to birth in the world, yet its infant mortality rates consistently are well above those of many European and developing countries where low-tech births are more common.

Nurse midwives generally use noninvasive techniques during delivery to aid labor in proceeding naturally while reducing the need for medical interventions. Midwives who assist at home births are available in some locations. If not, birthing centers and midwife services based in hospitals provide a good setting for women who would like to give birth naturally. For women with low-risk pregnancies, home births and birthing center births are equally as safe as hospital births and generally entail fewer invasive medical procedures.

Talking with Your Doctor

Whether you are talking to a fertility specialist, obstetrician, or midwife, it is vital to seek out health care practitioners you feel comfortable with. If you and your partner have not been able to conceive within a year, request that your doctor test both of you, as infertility problems are common in men as well as women. If you have had endometriosis, pelvic infections, sexually transmitted infections, pelvic pain, or surgery, or you are over thirty-five, have your doctor take a detailed health history from you (and your partner) after six months (rather than one year) of attempts with no conception, as your personal situation may create conditions that make it harder to conceive. Choose a physician who will give you the time you need to determine which treatments will be right for you.

If you have had miscarriages, find an OB/GYN who has worked with high-risk pregnancies. If you need additional support with grief from your pregnancy loss or assistance reducing anxiety during your pregnancy, ask your physician for recommendations of a therapist who regularly counsels women facing reproductive challenges.

Birth is an intimate experience, and you will have many prenatal visits, so it is helpful to select a care provider or group of providers whom you can trust. Partner with an obstetrician or midwife who will support your desire for an ideal birth experience. If you want to have a natural birth, interview health care providers about techniques they use to promote vaginal birth and choose a provider that will not push you toward a highly technical birth.

Interview fertility specialists to locate one whose team will provide emotional, psychological, and mind-body support to help enhance all assisted reproductive technologies.

Holistic Approaches to Conception, Pregnancy, and Birth

Integrative healing traditions encourage women to connect with the power of nature to expand the energy of fertility into their own lives. Holistic health modalities focus on creating a nourishing environment for the embryo through nutrition, movement, and mind-body balance. This approach concentrates on healing the endocrine system and releasing all toxicity, inflammation, and stagnant energy from the uterus.

Recent scientific knowledge emphasizes the benefits of slowing down and lowering stress for women who want to have a child. Fertility, pregnancy, and birth are powerful forms of creativity. If you have ever tried to write or make something artistic while under stress, you know that stress obstructs creativity. Similarly, high levels of stress can impede fertility and pregnancy and make giving birth more challenging. The strategies in this chapter provide stress-reduction tools that you can use to enhance fertility and pregnancy and create ease through birth, post-partum, and beyond.

Nutrition, Supplements, and Herbs

The uterine lining and the placenta supply all of the nutrients for the developing fetus, and the uterine muscles provide the power to release the baby during birth. It is important to obtain a full range of essential nutrients to prepare your uterus for conception, pregnancy, and birth. Use the nutrition plan in chapter four to enrich the uterus and ovaries. Eat a whole-foods diet rich in vitamins, minerals, essential fatty acids, and protein to regulate blood sugar. Reduce sugar, refined foods, caffeine, alcohol, and nicotine as much as possible.

Make sure you get plenty of healthy fats to develop high-quality eggs and nourish the ovaries and uterus. Take flax oil or eat ground flaxseeds to make sure you get ample omega-3 intake while trying to conceive to help regulate ovulation. Maintain flax supplementation during pregnancy. Decrease your fish intake and take krill or fish oil supplements, which have been found to have low mercury levels.[1] Continue during pregnancy, since fish oil supplementation has been shown to prevent miscarriage in at-risk women.[2] Eat calcium- and magnesium-rich foods throughout pregnancy, and take calcium and magnesium supplements if needed to provide the uterine muscles with plenty of energy for the birth process. Discuss all supplements with your health care provider during pregnancy to ensure the proper dosage for your specific needs.

If you and your partner are having difficulties conceiving or have had miscarriages, eliminating cigarettes, nicotine, caffeine, alcohol, drugs, and exposure to cigarette smoke will support your reproductive system and increase the health of both sperm and eggs. Acupuncture treatments can help people quit smoking naturally. Many acupuncturists offer weekly clinics for smoking cessation at a reduced rate.

Impaired fertility can be influenced by weight. If you are overweight, work with a nutritional counselor to make a whole-foods nutritional plan that you can combine with regular moderate exercise to help you gradually release weight and regulate ovulation. Some women with infertility problems are underweight, with a history of eating disorders or overexercise. If you need to increase your body weight to jump-start ovulation, moderate your exercise and seek help from a qualified therapist.

Do not diet during pregnancy or while breast-feeding. Instead, eat plenty of nutritious foods to ensure healthy weight gain and nourishment for you and your baby. Eat iron-rich foods such as garbanzo beans, green leafy vegetables, and blackstrap molasses. To help prevent pregnancy sickness, eat snacks and small meals throughout the day, including right before bed. To help avoid morning nausea, keep brown rice cakes or whole-grain crackers next to your bed to eat upon waking in the morning. Use a moderate amount of salt to help prevent preeclampsia, a sudden rise in high blood pressure accompanied by swelling and protein in the urine that can occur during the third trimester. Also called toxemia, preeclampsia can endanger both mother and child.

If you develop gestational diabetes while pregnant, modify your nutrition plan by reducing your intake of fruit and whole grains and eliminating all refined foods such as refined flours and sugar. Use the breathing, visualization, and cognitive restructuring techniques in chapter three to help reduce stress and balance insulin levels. Consult whole-foods cookbooks or work with a naturopath or holistic nutritionist to develop meal plans you can follow to keep your blood sugar levels in the healthy range.

Antioxidants can enhance fertility and lower the risk of miscarriage. To promote high-quality sperm and eggs and enrich the uterine lining for conception, take a good multimineral and multivitamin and encourage your partner to as well for several months before you start trying to conceive. Research shows that additional vitamin and mineral supplementation, including folic acid, B_6, B_{12}, zinc, vitamin C, vitamin E, and magnesium, can help couples who have experienced impaired fertility conceive.

Once you know you are pregnant, consult your health care provider to determine which prenatal vitamin is best for you. Additionally, taking probiotics throughout pregnancy provides beneficial intestinal bacteria for you and your developing baby. Using probiotics from the first trimester of pregnancy reduces infant allergies, eczema, and colic and gives your baby many advantages similar to those gained by breast-feeding. Probiotics also help prevent premature labor and encourage postpartum maternal weight loss.

Herbs have been used for thousands of years to treat infertility and prevent miscarriage. Red raspberry, false unicorn, chaste tree, black cohosh, and red clover boost fertility and aid conception. Red raspberry encourages the fertilized egg to implant and remain affixed to the endometrium. False unicorn works by regulating estrogen levels and strengthening the uterine lining. Chaste tree and black cohosh help decrease follicle-stimulating hormone (FSH) and increase progesterone naturally. Red clover balances estrogen and detoxifies the blood, but it can thin the blood. Do not use red clover before or after surgery or if you have a blood disorder.

For miscarriage prevention, use red raspberry, false unicorn, dong quai, and crampbark to prepare for pregnancy. Red raspberry, false unicorn, and crampbark inhibit miscarriage by relaxing and toning the uterus. Dong quai balances hormones and strengthens the uterus. Because dong quai and crampbark are not safe to take while pregnant, use these herbs only before conception to tone the uterus. Red raspberry can also reduce pregnancy sickness.

Always follow the directions on the package and take the recommended dosage. Discontinue most herbs if you think or confirm that you have conceived, unless an herbalist or health care provider recommends continuing herbs such as red raspberry, chaste tree, or false unicorn. Some naturopaths recommend continuing chaste tree during the first trimester and then tapering off slowly during the second trimester to prevent a sudden drop in progesterone and risk of miscarriage. Even though some medicinal herbs can be potentially unsafe during pregnancy, eating small amounts of food herbs such as garlic is safe. Do not self-diagnose during pregnancy. Always consult your midwife, physician, naturopath, or herbalist.

Movement and Bodywork

Uterine and pelvic position is important for conception, pregnancy, and birth. If your pelvis is tipped back from slouching, riding in cars, or sitting with a rounded spine, your uterus may be out of alignment. A misaligned uterus can cause difficulties conceiving, back pain during pregnancy, and challenges during birth. Follow the postural and movement guidelines in chapter five to sit and move in ways that encourage healthy uterine alignment.

Good posture combined with a daily practice of yoga positions such as cat (*marjaryasana*) and cow (*bitilasana*) poses and yogic squats will align the pelvic organs, enhance nervous system function, and increase blood flow to the uterus, ovaries, and fallopian tubes to optimize fertility. If you experience impaired fertility, ask your doctor during a routine visit to check your uterine position. Seek help from a physical therapist, chiropractor, or other bodyworker if you need additional assistance bringing your spine, pelvis, and uterus into balance. Visualize your uterus moving into perfect position while you exercise or undergo physical adjustments and imagine that your entire pelvic area is in complete harmony.

Deep tissue bodywork and massage can release scar tissue and heal the adhesions on the pelvic organs that are responsible for more than one-third of all infertility. Physical therapy techniques have been found to improve fertility in previously infertile women, including those with endometriosis.[3] Acupuncture can also help increase fertility naturally or as a complement to IVF. Acupuncture and chiropractic treatments can improve ovarian function and decrease uterine contractions. Acupuncture and other forms of energy work can regulate hormones, decrease stress, and reduce the side effects of fertility drugs. Before you begin IVF, prepare with the mind-body health treatments and self-care strategies in this book. Practice moderate exercise and postpone all serious athletic activity or training during IVF treatments.

During pregnancy, walking, swimming the breaststroke or crawl, and cat and cow poses along with modified squats can be practiced regularly to decrease back pain and get your baby in good position for an easier, less painful birth. Prenatal yoga is a great way to safely balance your body while gently increasing your flexibility. Avoid inversions and deep yoga squats during pregnancy. Daily movement and stretching improves mobility during the last trimester. I followed these practices before the birth of my son and had a relatively easy labor with no back pain or a need for pain medication. They are not guaranteed to be effective for every woman, but they are certainly worth trying.

Strengthen your pelvic floor by doing Kegel exercises (described in chapter five) daily, whether you plan to give birth vaginally or with a cesarean. Pressure on pelvic floor muscles during pregnancy can contribute to incontinence and pelvic organ prolapse postpartum and later in life, regardless of the delivery method. Research in Norway with three hundred women found that regular pelvic floor exercise during pregnancy facilitates and hastens labor and gives pregnant women more bladder control.[4]

In *Sit Up and Take Notice: Positioning Yourself for a Better Birth*, New Zealand midwife Pauline Scott shows how proper pelvic alignment encourages babies to move into the left anterior position with head down, facing backward on the left side of the uterus during the third trimester when space becomes tight.[5] Left anterior position creates less pressure and pain in the mother's back and facilitates easier movement through the birth canal. During your last trimester, be sure to ask your health care provider to inform you about your baby's position in the uterus. Along with doing the exercises in this section, rest on your left side frequently and cross your legs as little as possible. If your baby is facing forward in posterior position or head up in breech position, seek the help of a chiropractor or acupuncturist to safely turn the baby naturally in utero with no adverse effects. Numerous studies confirm the success and safety of the Webster technique, used by chiropractors, as well as acupuncture to promote optimal fetal positioning. If you are pregnant, always consult an acupuncturist before using self-acupressure.

Conscious Breathing

Nicole came to a workshop I gave on stress reduction for women. At the first session, we took a few minutes for the participants to talk about the stressors they were experiencing in their lives. As Nicole started to speak, tears welled up in her eyes. She shared that she was so overwhelmed by stress that she didn't even want to think about reducing it, but a friend had begged her to attend the event. The workshop included a half hour during which I taught participants how to use conscious breathing to release stress, pressure, and anxiety. At the end of the breathing segment, Nicole revealed that she was able to focus on her breath and release the constant onslaught of thoughts that had barraged her for as long as she could remember.

The next week, Nicole came to see me for a private consultation. When she came into my office I honestly didn't recognize her. Instead of the tense person with pain that was visible to anyone who paid attention, Nicole looked as if she had just spent a week at the beach. Nicole told me that she was about to try IVF for her second time and had been almost consumed by the fear of a possible failure for more than a year. She was so pleased with the relief that deep breathing had provided her during the past week that she wanted to learn more ways to support herself.

I helped Nicole identify beliefs that were creating her pain and also encouraged her to combine breathing with visualization and journaling to transform her inner landscape. She followed the Optimal Uterine Health Plan and consulted with her fertility specialist to understand each step of the IVF process so she could envision it working perfectly.

She practiced deep breathing with guided imagery for twenty minutes twice a day, imagining a healthy pregnancy and enjoying motherhood. Whenever she became stressed, she took the time to consciously connect with her breath and relax. This time IVF worked. Nicole gave birth to a beautiful baby girl.

Like Nicole, you can draw on conscious breathing to facilitate every stage of fertility, pregnancy, and birth. If you would like to conceive, practice the uterine breathing technique in chapter three to create a welcoming home for your baby. Breathe in love and light and breathe out stress and fear. Let go of doubt with every exhalation; breathe in your creative power as a woman. Inhale nourishment into the uterus and rich energy to the uterine lining. Breathe harmony and balance to the ovaries and pituitary gland.

Use these same techniques during pregnancy, nourishing yourself and your baby by breathing deeply into your uterus for several minutes each day. Employ conscious breathing to release apprehension about miscarriage as well as during any anxiety-producing health care procedures or appointments. Practice conscious breathing for fifteen minutes each day to help balance blood pressure and prevent preeclampsia.

Deep breathing reduces stress and can help regulate insulin levels during pregnancy. One client who had gestational diabetes found that her glucose numbers were noticeably lower on days she practiced deep breathing. She combined conscious breathing with guided imagery and a whole-foods diet daily for the rest of her pregnancy to decrease her blood sugar levels naturally.

Conscious breathing is an excellent tool that can make the entire birthing process more enjoyable and less painful or fearful. It can also help restore energy during postpartum: let your newborn baby's breathing remind you to relax and allow yourself to receive as much rejuvenating energy as possible with each breath.

Cognitive Restructuring

Many of us learn from society or our families that to be good mothers, women have to sacrifice their personal fulfillment and career success. Negative beliefs about the effects of motherhood on your personal freedom, career advancement, or your relationship with your life partner can create high stress and challenges with conception, pregnancy, birth, and postpartum. Women who have miscarriages and fertility problems generally experience elevated stress levels that can hinder future attempts to achieve a healthy pregnancy. Stress reduction is an effective tool to improve fertility naturally or as a complement to fertility treatments.

Use cognitive restructuring exercises to help you identify and change any attitudes that increase your stress and create fear about motherhood, having another child, pregnancy, giving birth, or not being able to have a biological child. It's now more common for women in their late thirties and forties to become pregnant and give birth. Know that it is possible to live a fulfilling life both personally and professionally as a mother and that millions of women become mothers through medical technologies, holistic fertility treatments, and adoption. Remember that you do not have to repeat nonnourishing family patterns in your own life or create limits based on antiquated and sexist social norms.

If you would like to experience natural birth but are constantly told that it is next to impossible, take a good natural childbirth class and ask any support people who will be present during the delivery to examine their own cultural attitudes about the birth process and create an environment in which you will be nurtured, honored, and pampered. Focus on how you can feel the most pleasure possible during birth. Hundreds of millions of women birth their babies without pain medication every year. However, be flexible if your delivery does require medical intervention. Medical technology can be a blessing if a true emergency does arise.

Pay attention to the language you use to talk about fertility, pregnancy, birth, and motherhood. Do you downplay your capability to become a mother to others because of your age? Is your language dark or pessimistic? If so, what would it be like to speak in a way that affirms your ability to become a mother and experience pregnancy and birth in a way that you desire? If you feel fear when speaking about your desires to become a mother, be pregnant, or give birth, use the journaling exercise that follows to reveal any attitudes you have that create this emotional response in your body.

Use journaling to explore any beliefs about pregnancy, birth, and motherhood you may hold. Write about your excitement and fears surrounding pregnancy, giving birth, and becoming a mother. Journal on the messages you have heard about pregnancy, birth, motherhood, miscarriage, or infertility from family, friends, health care providers, or society. Write all of your concerns about the ways in which being pregnant, giving birth, becoming a mother, or not being able to have biological children will affect your identity, body, lifestyle, career, or your relationship with your partner. Allow yourself to feel your feelings while you let any unacknowledged or repressed attitudes flow onto the paper. Do the "Four Steps to Change" in chapter three to transform any unsupportive and limiting beliefs and find new, powerful ways from which to view your life.

If you have experienced infertility problems or miscarriage, it is extremely important to allow yourself the emotional space to process any grief, anger, shame, and feelings of betrayal you may experience. After I had my miscarriage, I noticed the lack of social support available in our culture to help women deal with fertility problems or recover from miscarriage. As I looked for healthy ways to heal, I discovered that the Japanese commemorate miscarriages and abortions with shrines to

High maternal stress during pregnancy lowers infants' immune function and increases risks for asthma and allergies. Reducing stress will help ease conception, pregnancy, and birth, and promote health for your baby.

the unborn that are found in temples, on street corners, and in individual homes. Rather than being depressing, isolating places, the *mizuko kuyo* shrines are full of life and frequently visited by families who have lost children during pregnancy. The public shrines are often decorated with toys and have playgrounds so people can come to observe a moment of silence for their miscarried or aborted child while other children play and celebrate the exuberance of life.

You deserve to fully honor your loss whether it is caused by the emotional pain of not being able to become pregnant or from miscarriage. If you have impaired fertility or have had miscarriages, journal about your experiences to help you fully feel your emotions and uncover any judgmental and nonnourishing beliefs that you may hold about yourself and your situation. Use the "Belief Transformation Visualization and Ritual" in chapter eleven to open up to self-forgiveness and establish new beliefs that support you in your life and help you create healthy ways to connect with your body.

Seek help; do not isolate yourself. Talk about your feelings with supportive family members, friends, and a counselor or healer. Join a support group in your community or online. See whether it would be helpful to create a personal ritual to honor your loss and your mourning process so you can eventually open up to the future with as much ease as possible. If you have had an abortion and feel any guilt, self-judgment, or unresolved emotions about your choice, use these same processes to heal.

Visualization

Use the general visualization guidelines in chapter three to increase fertility, create a vibrant pregnancy, and have a joyous birth and postpartum experience. Allow yourself to fully connect with feelings of pleasure, peace, and power about becoming pregnant, bringing your child(ren) into the world, and being a mother.

Visualization for Fertility, Pregnancy, and Birth: Begin by closing your eyes and taking a few deep breaths. Relax your body by letting go of all tension and focusing your consciousness on your breath. Sense that your uterus is well nourished and that your ovaries, fallopian tubes, and entire endocrine system are in perfect harmony. Imagine that your eggs are strong and plentiful. See a healthy egg moving into your fallopian tube, where it joins with the right sperm to form the zygote. Feel the zygote effortlessly traveling through the tube into the uterus. Picture your uterus being able to easily implant the embryo and carry a healthy pregnancy to term. Envision your pregnancy as happy, fun, and easy.

Imagine effortlessly giving birth, assisted by talented health care providers and loving family and friends. Feel your excitement when you birth a beautiful, healthy baby. Envisage motherhood as being full of freedom, support, love, and grace. Go ahead and let yourself visualize your most wonderful future as a mother, with family life and career flowing in perfect balance. Sense all the fun and growth you will have with your child(ren).

Employ guided imagery to boost any fertility treatments you may undergo. Picture technologies working perfectly and your body easily receiving the treatments, producing and implanting healthy egg(s), and remaining pregnant. If you notice that you visualize unsuccessful outcomes or an unhappy future when you think about fertility treatments, pregnancy, or motherhood, use the cognitive restructuring exercises detailed earlier to heal the beliefs inside you that are generating a dark future.

Nurture Creativity

Traditional Chinese medicine recommends strengthening your bond with natural and cosmic energy to enhance fertility and pregnancy. To connect with the creative power of nature, work in a garden, take a walk in the woods, or just spend time relaxing outdoors. Gaze at the stars and moon at night; soak up sunlight for at least twenty minutes every day.

Immerse yourself in creative energy by expanding your creativity in ways that truly bring you pleasure. Surround yourself with or read about innovative people and ideas that inspire you. Think about how enhancing your nutrition, movement, beliefs, breathing practices, and vision for the future will help develop the fertile conditions so necessary for conception and healthy pregnancy. Engage in fun-filled, expressive activities such as painting, singing, dancing, cooking, or writing to amplify the creative power in your life. Envision your life being enriched by motherhood and also celebrate yourself for who you are right now, feeling gratitude for all the good things you have already created for yourself.

CHAPTER TEN

Menopause

The time of transition known as menopause has been honored by societies throughout the world. For millennia in many indigenous cultures, menopausal women have been recognized as political, economic, and spiritual leaders. However, in the West, menopause has generally been viewed as a difficult and even debilitating time of life.

During the previous century, while biomedical researchers defined menopause as a deficiency disease, women's health advocates challenged the use of such a negative designation for a normal stage of women's lives. Feminist scholars and holistic health practitioners maintain that menopause is an emotional and physiological transformational process that can help women open up to immense power and personal growth. From a mind-body perspective, the physiological changes during menopause that end both the capacity for reproduction and monthly hormonal fluctuations create space for new energy, vision, and focus in women's lives. With this growth, opportunities open for women to develop their wisdom, creativity, and true desires like never before.

From a medical point of view, the menopause transition is divided into several stages. Menopause is defined as one year with no menstruation following a woman's last menses, unless it is surgically induced by removal of both ovaries, in which case menopause begins immediately. Postmenopause refers to the remainder of a woman's life after her last menstrual period. Perimenopause is the life stage immediately preceding menopause, when a woman experiences changes in her menstrual cycle. Premenopause describes the phase of a woman's life from menarche to menopause. Temporary menopause may also be caused by a variety of medications used for endometriosis, fibroids, or cancer that disrupt ovarian function and inhibit menstruation.

This terminology can be confusing, as women will not know which menses will be their last unless menopause is surgically induced. Additionally, Western women frequently experience a wide variety of physiological and emotional symptoms during perimenopause that extend into the early years of postmenopause. So most women's lived experiences are not accurately represented by these fairly rigidly defined categories. To simplify, at times I will use the term "menopause transition" to signify this multifaceted process that occurs in women's lives.

By 2020, there will be nearly one billion menopausal women in the world. The average age of menopause for American women is fifty-one. In the United States, perimenopause generally begins in the mid- to late forties and lasts five to seven years. For a small percentage of Western women, perimenopause begins in the late thirties or early forties and continues for more than a decade. In non-Western cultures some women go through menopause in their late thirties and forties without experiencing the perimenopausal stage. Instead, they may simply not resume menstruation after breast-feeding their last child. Yet more than 80 percent of Western women experience symptoms during perimenopause such as erratic menstrual cycles, hot flashes, sleep disturbances, night sweats, vaginal dryness, depression, mood swings, and difficulties concentrating.

Medical anthropology studies illustrate that challenging symptoms are not an inevitable consequence of menopause. Mayan women in Mexico and Rajput women in India describe having no menopausal symptoms at all. Filipino women frequently do not associate physiological problems with menopause. Instead, they tend to consider menopause as a transition that ushers in positive changes such as increased energy, better moods, and improved sex. Women in many African and Native American societies welcome menopause into their lives because of the wisdom, clarity, and insight they believe it brings.

Even without long-term estrogen therapies, postmenopausal women in many developing societies have much lower rates of osteoporosis and heart disease than women in the West. They eat mostly plant-based diets, are more physically active, and live in cultures that reinforce positive outlooks on menopause and aging—and thus have little need to resort to all the medications so commonly prescribed to menopausal women in the United States. The lifestyle changes and holistic health modalities in this book can assist you in creating ease during your own menopausal process, no matter where you live. Follow the mind-body practices to help prevent and alleviate physical and emotional symptoms and make perimenopause and postmenopause enjoyable life phases full of creativity, freedom, and wellness.

Biomedical Approaches to Perimenopause and Menopause

To determine menopausal status, many biomedical physicians will test follicle-stimulating hormone (FSH) levels to determine whether the ovaries have stopped ovulatory activity. High FSH levels can determine whether ovulation has stopped, but testing for FSH does not detect blood estrogen levels. FSH levels can fluctuate significantly during perimenopause, so it may not always be an accurate test if hormone levels are still in flux.

Until very recently, the biomedical approach to menopause involved encouraging virtually all healthy postmenopausal women to take hormones for the rest of their lives to prevent uncomfortable menopausal symptoms, heart disease, and osteoporosis, despite the absence of long-term studies confirming the safety or efficacy of continuous estrogen supplementation. This protocol combined estrogen with progestin in hormone replacement therapy (HRT) to prevent uterine cancer, or, for women who had undergone hysterectomies, used estrogen therapy (ET) alone. In the last decade several important studies revealed that estrogen and hormone replacement therapies used longer than five years can increase risks of stroke, heart attack, breast cancer, blood clots, Alzheimer's, and dementia, especially if used later in life or started five years or more after menopause.

HRT is still given for less than five years to relieve menopausal-related vaginal problems and vasomotor symptoms such as hot flashes, night sweats, and sleep disturbances. Hormonal therapy alleviates more than 70 percent of all vasomotor symptoms. HRT may be prescribed as a topical cream for vaginal dryness and thinning in women who do not wish to use it for other types of symptom reduction.

For osteoporosis, HRT may be used for women who do not tolerate nonhormonal drugs, such as Fosamax or Boniva, which can damage the gastrointestinal tract. Some medical practitioners still advocate administering HRT during perimenopause to treat depression or prevent heart disease, but most experts do not recommend this. In addition to the potential serious health risks already discussed, HRT may cause side effects such as breast tenderness, bloating, and nausea.

Many of the symptoms previously attributed to low estrogen levels by biomedical practitioners—such as anxiety, depression, reduced libido, cognitive difficulties, incontinence, weight gain, joint pain, and fatigue— are now thought to be associated more generally with aging. However, in some cases, these conditions may be caused by menopausal difficulties (for example, vaginal dryness may create less interest in sex, or mood swings and anxiety may result from sleep disturbances). There are a variety of medical treatments that physicians can use to treat these conditions in lieu of HRT; however, most doctors simply focus on symptom reduction rather than addressing underlying imbalances.

Talking with Your Doctor

Despite conventional medical thinking, many women do not have drastically low estrogen levels after menopause, because there are other sources of estrogen, such as body fat, estrogen-rich diets, and environmental estrogens. Even though the ovaries lower their production of estrogen after menopause, the body continues to produce many other important hormones, such as testosterone and dehydroepiandrosterone (DHEA) in the adrenal glands, the pineal gland, fat cells, and elsewhere, which can convert into moderate levels of estrogen. Before beginning estrogen therapy, request a blood analysis to determine your blood hormone levels. Some women have plenty of estrogen, but may be depleted of progesterone, testosterone, or DHEA.

Talk to a knowledgeable doctor about the benefits of using bioidentical hormones rather than standard hormone replacement. Bioidentical hormones include estrogens, progesterone, DHEA, and testosterone. Bioidentical hormones match the same chemical structure of the hormones that your body naturally produces. Many physicians believe that bioidentical hormones more closely mimic the hormones the body naturally produces after menopause, are metabolized easier, and have fewer risks. Women frequently experience symptom reduction and increased vitality from tiny amounts of one or more bioidentical hormones, such as progesterone or DHEA. However, there are no long-term studies of the safety or efficacy of bioidentical hormones.

Stay on hormones for the shortest period possible and use the nutritional recommendations in this book to support your body while on medications. The ovaries continue to work in concert with the adrenals to produce important hormones after menopause, so if you do have a hysterectomy, keep your ovaries if possible. If you have had your ovaries

If you do choose to take standard or bioidentical hormones, have your medical practitioner evaluate your personal risks before beginning therapy.

- Ask your care provider to conduct a full health assessment, including a mammogram, physical, and oral health history before beginning any hormone therapy.
- Include a bone density scan if you are using hormones to prevent osteoporosis.
- Work with your physician to determine the lowest dose you can take that still delivers effective results.

removed and feel the need for continuous hormonal replacement, work with an experienced physician and pharmacist who can help you determine acceptable low levels of hormones for long-term use.

Address conditions such as incontinence and vaginal dryness with your health care provider as soon as they occur. There are many available treatment options used to reduce these common symptoms that your doctor can offer you, such as biofeedback or surgery for incontinence or topical hormones for vaginal issues. The sooner you bring up these concerns, the easier it will be to treat them.

Holistic Approaches to Perimenopause and Menopause

Rather than a deficiency disease, holistic traditions consider menopause a transformational process that encourages women to take stock of their lives and examine their hopes, dreams, and expectations of who they truly are and what they want in the next stage of life. Like all rites of passage, menopause takes one's life and magnifies it under a lens. Life satisfaction, career goals, and relationships all come under deep scrutiny to be explored and reconfigured in ways not thought possible before.

From a mind-body perspective, challenging symptoms during the menopause transition are the body's way of communicating that it needs increased nourishment and support. Along with signifying depletion or stagnation in the endocrine system, blood, liver, or kidneys, physical symptoms can be caused by emotional, energetic, and spiritual imbalances. Research shows that menopause symptoms are related to stress levels, lifestyle, and attitudes about menopause and aging. Make yourself your first priority and use my nutritional, exercise, and stress-reduction suggestions to create vibrancy during peri- and postmenopause.

Nutrition, Supplements, and Herbs

Combine the following recommendations with the nutrition plan in chapter four to achieve optimal health during your entire menopausal transition. This eating plan will help improve your endocrine function and provide symptom relief during perimenopause. It will also help prevent heart disease and osteoporosis as you age.

As I discussed in chapter four, most Western women get more dietary calcium than women in developing countries, yet we have much higher rates of osteoporosis because our diets and lifestyles cause us to secrete calcium at higher rates as well. A 2003 study at Oklahoma State University demonstrated that women not on HRT who consumed soy protein lost less calcium and developed stronger bones than women who took a milk-based protein.[1] To reduce calcium loss and promote new bone tissue growth through nutrition, eat a plant-based diet with plenty of leafy green vegetables, essential fatty acids, minerals from foods, and supplements. Get vitamin D from sunshine daily if possible, and decrease animal protein consumption, soft drinks, cigarettes, caffeine, alcohol, saturated and trans fats, and salt.

For perimenopause symptom relief, increase your estrogen levels naturally through intake of healthy phytoestrogens such as fresh fruits, vegetables, ground flaxseeds, and soy foods, such as tofu and tempeh. There are some cautions about soy; if you have limited thyroid function, take thyroid medicine, have a history of breast cancer, or take tamoxifen, talk to your health care provider to determine safe soy consumption levels. To alleviate hot flashes, eliminate alcohol, cigarettes, spicy foods, and caffeine, including regular and decaf coffee, soft drinks, and chocolate. Use evening primrose oil to help prevent premenstrual breast swelling and pain during perimenopause. Natural vitamin E can help decrease hot flashes, particularly at high levels such as 800 to 1,000 mg/day. Work with your doctor to find the correct dose for you, particularly if you are diabetic.

Take a multimineral and a multivitamin to get the appropriate levels of B, E, D, and C vitamins, and manganese, boron, and magnesium. To support your adrenal and pineal glands and encourage your body's continued production of sufficient hormones naturally, refrain from refined carbohydrates (starches and sweets) and get plenty of B vitamins. To ease sleep disturbances, try melatonin.

Herbs can reduce symptoms and promote wellness during every stage of menopause when used for several months or longer. Black cohosh, red clover, and dong quai can help relieve a number of vasomotor symptoms such as hot flashes, night sweats, and sleep disorders. However, do not use dong quai if you are regularly experiencing heavy bleeding or while menstruating. Wild yam and chaste tree encourage progesterone production and help balance irregular menses, ease heavy bleeding during perimenopause, and alleviate many other menopausal symptoms. Wild yam cream assists in restoring vaginal tissue naturally. Dandelion and milk thistle will strengthen your liver and help with hormone metabolization. Ginkgo can be used to enhance cognition and correct memory problems. St. John's wort is frequently effective in relieving depression and restoring a sense of emotional well-being.

Movement and Bodywork

Follow the general exercise recommendations in chapter five to help yourself feel your best throughout the entire menopause process and beyond. In addition to getting at least thirty minutes of aerobic exercise four times each week, during the menopausal years it's particularly important to continue or begin weight training and weight-bearing exercises that engage the upper and lower body to help encourage bone growth and prevent osteoporosis. Despite previous biomedical theories, women can develop new bone tissue even after estrogen levels lower, so focus on strength training at least three times each week to maintain and strengthen your body.

Yoga and Pilates can help you improve your posture, develop flexibility, and prevent vertebral compression. Yoga has also been shown to help women manage menopausal symptoms.[2] Focus on poses that help you open your heart, lengthen your spine, and increase mobility in your hips. If you have any joint problems or injuries, let your yoga or Pilates instructor know before class so she or he can provide you with alternative poses that are safe. Use the Kegel exercises described in chapter five daily to help maintain your pelvic core strength and prevent incontinence.

If you experience hot flashes during strenuous exercise, reduce the intensity of your routine while you increase the duration, so you still get the calorie-burning benefits you have been used to. Alternatively, you may want to try swimming and water aerobics, both of which can help you remain cool and provide you with excellent aerobic benefits while being gentle on the joints. However, it is important to combine water exercises with plenty of weight-bearing activities to strengthen your bones.

Homeopathy, acupressure, conscious breathing, acupuncture, reflexology, and other energy work modalities such as Reiki and Healing Touch can help reduce menopausal discomforts and strengthen the body. If you want to use self-care techniques, research shows that a simple foot massage as described in chapter five administered regularly may be almost as effective as reflexology in reducing psychological symptoms, hot flashes, and night sweats during menopause.[3] Any practices that induce relaxation such as aromatherapy or sound therapy help ease a wide range of menopausal symptoms.

Conscious Breathing

Deep breathing relaxes the body, releases stress, and decreases hot flash intensity and frequency. Conscious breathing is a wonderful way to enhance your pituitary, hypothalamus, adrenals, thyroid, and other endocrine glands, so vital to health during menopause. My clients have used the following breathing exercise to ease multiple menopausal symptoms and nourish other stages of uterine health. This exercise guides you to consciously concentrate your breathing on your endocrine glands one by one. Breathe into each gland as outlined here for a minute or more. Note: I suggest receiving and releasing certain qualities during this practice; if you are moved to focus on different energy, please follow your inner guidance.

Endocrine Restoration Breathing Exercise: Using the breathing instructions in chapter three, find a quiet place where you can relax. Begin by breathing deeply through your mouth and imagine yourself breathing into all of your cells, muscles, organs, and bones. Allow yourself to receive several breaths like this, enjoying the opportunity to breathe more fully into your belly, back, shoulders, and torso. Visualize breathing down into your legs and feet.

Begin to focus on your endocrine system by breathing into the pituitary gland, which is located in a small bony cavity at the base of the brain. The pituitary produces several important hormones that affect thyroid, adrenal, and ovarian function. During menopause the pituitary becomes very active, producing large amounts of luteinizing hormone (LH) and FSH in an attempt to restart the ovaries. For a minute or more, breathe ease and nourishment to the pituitary. Intend that your inhalations relax, revitalize, and balance the pituitary as your exhalations let go of overexertion, heat, fatigue, and struggle.

During your next breaths, turn your attention to the hypothalamus, which is located above the pituitary in the central part of the brain. The hypothalamus acts as the body's thermostat and secretes hormones to regulate pituitary and endocrine function. Breathe in cool, stabilizing energy to the hypothalamus. Imagine that with each inhale your hypothalamus receives joy, peace, love, and wisdom and is able to keep your endocrine system and body temperature operating in perfect balance and harmony. Imagine that your exhalations release confusion, dysfunction, and tiredness.

Focus your awareness on the pineal gland, which is also found in the middle of the brain. The tiny pineal regulates aging and produces melatonin, the anti-aging hormone that also assists in balancing sleep cycles and stabilizing mood. Breathe in balance, rhythm, flow, abundance, clarity, and insight to the pineal. As you breathe out, release chaos, depletion, hardness, disconnection, and all blocks out of the pineal gland.

Next, direct your breath to the thyroid and parathyroid glands, which are located in the neck. The thyroid produces hormones that regulate how quickly chemical reactions occur in the body, including how quickly cells produce energy from food, while the parathyroid glands influence blood calcium levels. If the thyroid is not fully functioning, you will experience weight gain, fatigue, and food cravings. Breathe in ease, grace, and equilibrium into the thyroid glands, and with every exhalation, release stuck, rigid energy.

Move your breathing to the adrenal glands, which are located above the kidneys on the back of the torso. Along with helping you deal with stress, the adrenal glands produce more than one hundred other hormones, including androgens, such as testosterone, and DHEA, which can be converted into estrogen. With every breath, receive renewal and rejuvenation in the adrenals and release fatigue and tiredness.

Shift your awareness to the ovaries, which continue to produce important hormones after menopause. Breathe in freedom, power, and creativity to the ovaries; with your exhales, release frustration, uselessness, and resentment. If you are in perimenopause and are undergoing fertility treatments to conceive, breathe in vitality and life to your ovaries and breathe out hopelessness, anger, and fear.

To prevent or reduce menopausal problems, do this exercise for twenty minutes once a day or for a few minutes several times throughout your day. If you have frequent hot flashes or night sweats, practice this breathing once during the day and again in the evening before bed to reduce night sweats and improve sleep patterns. Begin conscious breathing at the first sign of a hot flash to diminish intensity and duration.

Cognitive Restructuring

In Western societies women often view menopause as a time of loss of youth or femininity and a period of declining health. Women report fewer difficulties during menopause in cultures where attitudes about menopause and aging are positive. If you currently view menopause in a negative light, journal about what it would feel like to shift your perspective and experience menopause as a transformational process that provides remarkable opportunity for personal growth, wellness, and development.

Write about the changes that have occurred in your life and body during menopause, examining how you feel about the emotional and physical aspects of your transition. Journal on ways you can feel positive and nourish strong self-esteem and body image during menopause. Consider how your personal power and wisdom have increased and will continue to develop during your next stage of life. Write about any beneficial role models you can connect with to help make menopause a positive rite of passage in your own life.

Also contemplate how your relationships have changed during your menopausal transition. Connect with your inner knowledge to reveal strategies that will help you increase your fulfillment in relationships with your family and friends, including with a significant other or any children you have. Reflect on changes other than menopause that may be taking place in your life, such as career transitions, retirement preparation, caring for aging parents, children leaving home, the arrival of grandchildren, marriage, or divorce. Explore how these changes affect your stress levels, health, and your ability to fully care for yourself during menopause. Observe whether you hold any beliefs that increase your stress and prevent you from more fully enjoying your life, body, relationships, and work right now. Write about how it might feel to release these views and adopt healthier attitudes about your personal power, health, life, relationships, menopause, and aging that would help you create more fun and joy throughout your menopausal journey and beyond.

Visualization

Patricia was an accountant at a large firm. She entered into perimenopause in her early forties. She had a heavy workload that became almost unbearable for a few months each year, and at her busiest times, Patricia became plagued by hot flashes that lowered her productivity at work.

She came to me to develop tools to help handle the stress in her life that seemed to be triggering her menopausal symptoms.

In our work together, Patricia focused on transforming her negative beliefs about herself, her health, and her life, as well as her work situation. She gave up caffeine, began using herbs, and altered her diet to help balance her hormones. I guided Patricia to envisage cool, blue water flowing into her head, bringing her energy and sustenance and releasing stress and fear. I encouraged Patricia to really feel this nourishing clear water balancing and revitalizing her pituitary gland and hypothalamus, the area of the brain that regulates temperature.

Patricia focused on sensing this refreshing energy at least twice a day for fifteen minutes, accompanying her visualization with deep conscious breathing into her entire body. Within a few weeks, Patricia noticed that her hot flashes had decreased significantly. She found that if she skipped her practice for a few days because she felt too busy, the hot flashes would return. So during her most stressful months, she worked the visualization into her schedule to help support her mind and body.

Endocrine Gland Visualization: I have used this imagery to help many women reduce vasomotor symptoms. To do it, use the general guidelines for practicing visualization in chapter three and imagine the beautiful, sparkling water or a stream of golden light pouring into your head and streaming into your entire body. You may want to picture yourself standing under a gorgeous waterfall. Let yourself fully receive the restorative energy of the water or golden light. Allow it to flow into every cell of your body and cleanse your endocrine organs and glands completely.

To help relieve hot flashes, feel the water or golden energy rejuvenating and stabilizing your hypothalamus and pituitary. Let this refreshing imagery signal to your hypothalamus that you want your body to remain at a comfortable temperature at all times. Follow this visualization with the exercise in the preceding Conscious Breathing section. If you regularly experience night sweats, use this visualization before bed. This imagery is also excellent for alleviating headaches.

To maintain and restore wellness during the menopause transition, you may also want to visualize the endocrine glands discussed in the previous breathing exercise as vital and healthy. Picture the pituitary, hypothalamus, pineal, thyroid, adrenals, and ovaries vibrating beautifully with balanced energy and life. Sense that each endocrine gland constantly receives plenty of nourishment so that it can generate the perfect amounts of hormones for your body. Know that as you age, your glands, uterus, and ovaries will remain strong, vibrant, and full of power. Envision your entire endocrine system operating in perfect clarity and harmony.

Some scientists believe that overactivity of the pituitary may stimulate the hypothalamus and cause hot flashes and night sweats. Imagine that you can communicate with your pituitary gland and tell it that it doesn't have to work so hard, because you are moving on to the next phase of life in which your creative energy will not be focused on ovulation. Let the pituitary know that it can be in perfect balance and harmony for the rest of your life.

Envision the pineal producing a healthy abundance of the anti-aging hormone melatonin. Picture this ocean of melatonin flowing to each of your cells, rejuvenating your mind, brain, body, and spirit and helping you grow and age with ease and grace. If you regularly feel fatigue, imagine that your adrenals are healthy and whole. Feel nourishing energy flowing from nature to restore your adrenal glands.

Visualize vital golden energy streaming into your ovaries so they continue to produce plenty of hormones to support you during and after your menopause transition. Know your entire endocrine system is full of grace. Connect with your vagina and pelvic floor and imagine this area of your body coming into perfect harmony. See your life being full of pleasure and sexual energy. Imagine sex being fun and feeling good. Envisage yourself continually renewing your bone tissue and all of your bones becoming stronger and denser. Picture your spine growing longer and more flexible as you age. Imagine healthy, joyful aging filled with growth, love, and wisdom.

An Ancient Rite of Passage

Some biomedical practitioners have inaccurately claimed that menopause is an unnatural process for which women's bodies are unequipped, brought on by increased longevity in the past two centuries. This erroneous assumption came about from physicians incorrectly interpreting historical data. Virtually all historical and anthropological research proves that women have lived through menopause since the beginning of human history. In fact, anthropologists surmise that the skills, wisdom, and energy of menopausal women gave early humans the ability to prosper and thrive. This theory, known as the grandmother hypothesis, explains that without the support of postmenopausal females, our species would not have been able to evolve as successfully as we have. No longer occupied with childbearing, older females were able to invest their time teaching, protecting, and helping their children and grandchildren, which allowed more of our species to acquire the tools and education needed to survive and have children of their own.

Menopause is a normal stage of uterine health that has been made difficult by our modern lifestyles and societal biases. Just like the bodies of women in traditional societies, your body innately knows how to make the changes that occur during menopause—it just needs ample nourishment to do it with as much ease as possible. Whenever riding the wave of menopause feels tumultuous to you, connect to your inner wisdom to help make navigating this terrain easier. See whether viewing menopause as a positive growth process rather than a period of potential decline can help you expand your personal power, freedom, and wellness. Use self-care techniques to support your body, mind, and spirit throughout menopause as you usher in an exciting new stage of your life.

CHAPTER ELEVEN

Hysterectomy

Each year, six hundred thousand American women undergo a hysterectomy, the second most common surgery in the United States after cesarean section. Approximately 10 percent are performed for cancer and considered medically necessary. The other 90 percent are performed for benign conditions such as uterine fibroids, endometriosis, menstrual problems, and uterine prolapse, and they are usually elective.

For some women, having a hysterectomy brings relief and restores quality of life. Others experience a wide range of problematic symptoms after surgery, including pelvic pain, loss of sexual desire, urinary and bowel problems, depression, nerve impairment, weight gain, and postural pain. Hysterectomy can damage the blood supply and nerves to the ovaries, reducing ovarian function and causing premature menopause in some cases. Removing the uterus increases risks of high blood pressure and heart attack. Further, women who also have their ovaries removed during hysterectomy face additional elevated risks of heart disease, hip fracture, dementia, and stroke.

As I describe in chapter two, the uterus contributes to women's lifelong wellness even though many current biomedical providers may be unaware of its importance to our heart health, posture, and sexual enjoyment. Hysterectomy does serve as a lifesaving solution in cases of uterine and pelvic cancers. It can also help women suffering with severe problems from benign uterine conditions improve their quality of life. However, unnecessary hysterectomies are still commonly performed when less-invasive procedures would restore uterine health, because of the antiquated biases about the uterus held by some practitioners in the biomedical community.

If you have a benign uterine problem that is not life-threatening or debilitating, consider combining less-invasive medical treatment options discussed in earlier chapters with mind-body techniques to restore your uterine health without the risks of hysterectomy complications. If you have developed severe uterine issues and choose to have a hysterectomy, use the holistic techniques in this chapter and the Optimal Uterine Health Plan (part two) to achieve the best surgery and recovery outcomes possible. Whatever your choice, know that you can develop lifelong wellness through healthy nutrition, regular exercise, stress reduction, and other holistic health techniques.

Biomedical Approaches to Hysterectomy

In the United States, hysterectomies are most commonly performed on women aged thirty-five to forty-nine for uterine fibroids. Women between thirty and thirty-five most frequently have hysterectomies for endometriosis; those under thirty generally have hysterectomies for irregular menstruation or cervical dysplasia. Women fifty-five or older most commonly undergo hysterectomy for uterine prolapse or cancer. Biomedical experts surmise that many hysterectomies conducted in the United States for benign conditions are medically unnecessary.[1]

There are four main types of hysterectomy. Total hysterectomy removes the entire uterus and cervix. Subtotal or supracervical hysterectomy removes the entire uterus except the cervix. Radical hysterectomy removes the uterus including the cervix, the upper third of the vagina, pelvic lymph nodes, and the tissue surrounding the uterus, and is usually performed in cases of cancer. Simple hysterectomy removes the uterus and leaves the pelvic lymph nodes and tissue that surrounds the uterus.

Half of the six hundred thousand hysterectomies performed in the United States annually also include oophorectomy, the surgical removal of the ovaries. Removing the ovaries may increase women's risks of heart disease, stroke, osteoporosis, Parkinson's disease, and dementia because the ovaries continue to produce important hormones throughout a woman's life—if they are not surgically removed. A recent review of the research published in *Obstetrics & Gynecology* recommends that women who undergo hysterectomy for benign conditions who do not have an increased risk for ovarian cancer will protect their health if they retain their ovaries.[2] Additionally, salpingectomy, removal of the fallopian tubes, should be performed only if there is a valid reason.

The three main surgical approaches for hysterectomy are vaginal, abdominal, or laparoscopic. The uterus can be removed with traditional surgical procedures through the vagina or either a horizontal or a vertical incision in the abdomen. Hysterectomy can also be performed using a laparoscope, as described in chapter seven, during a vaginal procedure or when surgeons make very small incisions in the abdomen. In a press release dated October 21, 2009, the American College of Obstetricians and Gynecologists recommend vaginal hysterectomy as the safest procedure for benign conditions because vaginal hysterectomies generally have fewer complications and quicker recovery times.

Hysterectomy is generally medically necessary for uterine, cervical, and ovarian cancers. It is most frequently performed for benign conditions such as uterine fibroids, endometriosis, and uterine prolapse. Less-invasive surgical procedures and other treatment options for fibroids, endometriosis, and menstrual irregularities are discussed in the corresponding chapters. Always consult your health care provider if you experience irregular menstruation, and have an endometrial biopsy if endometrial hyperplasia or uterine cancer is suspected. Pap tests generally reveal precancerous cervical conditions before they pose a serious risk of developing into cervical cancer, so be sure to have yearly gynecological examinations and follow your doctor's recommendation for Pap test frequency depending on your health history, age, and level of risk.

If a Pap test detects low-grade cervical dysplasia, your doctor may recommend monitoring your condition and waiting to see if the dysplasia will go away on its own. With some abnormalities, your doctor may suggest having a colposcopy, a procedure that uses a special microscope called a colposcope to view the cervix and take a tissue sample to biopsy. If cancer or any invasive high-grade abnormalities are found, your doctor will most likely recommend hysterectomy. If the abnormalities are less serious and noninvasive and you would like to keep your uterus, your physician may offer a number of procedures that remove or destroy cervical tissue, in lieu of a hysterectomy.

The loop electrosurgical excision procedure (LEEP) removes any malignant tissue and the part of the cervix where more malignancy could develop. Cervical conization surgically removes a larger, cone-shaped area of tissue to prevent the possibility of future malignancy. Cryosurgery destroys precancerous and noninvasive cancerous cervical tissue by freezing it. Carbon dioxide laser vaporizes abnormal cervical tissue and leaves healthy tissue intact. If you have one of these procedures, your physician may recommend that you have Pap tests at more regular intervals.

If you have tested positive for a strain of human papilloma virus (HPV) that puts you at higher risk for cervical cancer, your care provider may recommend more frequent Pap tests.

Talking with Your Doctor

If you have a non–life-threatening uterine disorder, always ask your doctor to inform you of all available biomedical alternatives to hysterectomy. If your physician suggests that hysterectomy is medically necessary for a benign, non–life-threatening condition, get a second opinion to find out whether there are less-invasive options for you. In seeking a second opinion, do your homework and find a doctor you know is familiar with and open to alternatives.

If you decide it is necessary for you to have your uterus surgically removed, talk to your doctor about which type of hysterectomy will be best for your condition. If your cervix is healthy, have a subtotal or supracervical hysterectomy so you have fewer complications. Just like other areas of the uterus, the cervix produces prostaglandins that may have important effects on other areas of the body. Maintaining the cervix also promotes more sexual pleasure and anatomical support after hysterectomy. Even though removing healthy ovaries along with the uterus is a common practice, medical experts now advise against this in women with normal risk of ovarian cancer, because the ovaries play an important role in overall health after menopause. Unless you have ovarian disease or an elevated risk for ovarian cancer that you are concerned about, find a doctor who understands the long-term health benefits of retaining your ovaries. If you do have your ovaries removed, see the sections on bioidentical hormones and mind-body techniques in the previous chapter.

When talking to your surgeon about your hysterectomy, ask about possible risks, type of anesthesia, type of incision, length of surgery and recovery, and when you can resume exercise and work as well as sexual activity. Your physician will want to complete a full evaluation and a series of tests to confirm that you are ready for surgery.

Holistic Approaches to Hysterectomy

From the holistic health perspective, all parts of the body are important. Integrative medicine is based on the theory that everything in the body is connected, thus removing individual parts can have negative consequences for the whole. As I describe in chapter two, the uterus plays a meaningful role in the body beyond reproduction and may positively affect other body functions and areas in ways not currently understood by medical researchers.

True healing requires correcting all physical, emotional, and energetic imbalances that created the disease rather than just treating the symptoms. Even after a hysterectomy it is essential to restore the endo-crine, immune, and nervous systems, as well as the liver. It is equally important to balance the emotions and the body's energy. Whether you would like to avoid a hysterectomy or remain healthy after one, combin-ing the mind-body strategies in this chapter with those presented in the Optimal Uterine Health Plan (part two) will help you create lifelong wellness.

In an energy medicine framework, a hysterectomy removes part of the second chakra and in some instances can deplete the energies located there. If you do have a hysterectomy, use visualization, conscious breath-ing, and any methods that interest you to enhance creativity, sexuality, relationships, feminine energy, and personal power in your life.

Nutrition, Supplements, and Herbs

If you would like to try to prevent having a hysterectomy, follow the guidelines in chapter four as well as the nutrition suggestions in the chapter related to your uterine imbalance (endometriosis, fibroid, or menstrual difficulties). To help prevent cervical dysplasia and cervical cancer, eat plenty of yellow, red, orange, and dark green vegetables and fruits, such as tomatoes, carrots, winter squash, kale, parsley, collards, yellow pepper, watermelon, chard, and bok choy. Get plenty of dietary and supplemental vitamin A, B complex, C, fish oil, and lycopene.

If you decide to have a hysterectomy, continue the eating plan in chapter four along with the recommendations in this section for the rest of your life to provide your endocrine system with the nutrients you need to maintain lifelong wellness. Eat plenty of fiber-rich foods before your surgery; pain medicine generally makes the bowels sluggish for a

If you are diagnosed with cervical dysplasia, work with your phy-sician as well as a naturopath to prevent it from developing to a more serious stage or, in some cases, to help reverse it, with nutri-tion and supplements.

few days. For recovery after surgery, include fresh organic vegetable juice daily with the other eating recommendations in chapter four to help give your body the nutrients it needs to heal and reduce inflammation naturally.

Each day, eat plenty of tart cherries, to help reduce pain, and goji berries, blueberries, and raspberries to decrease inflammation. Drink plenty of water to help detoxify from the medications used with your surgery. Get plenty of fiber from organic vegetables and fruits, and avoid refined foods, dairy products, and other foods that can increase constipation during the recovery period. Take a good multimineral and multivitamin throughout your entire recovery.

A whole-foods diet that balances hormonal health can help improve libido after a hysterectomy. If you experience decreased sexual desire after your hysterectomy recovery, limit refined foods, sugars, and unhealthy fats, and get most of your calories from vegetables, legumes, whole grains, fruits, healthy fats, and plant-based proteins. Always have a good breakfast and eat several small meals throughout the day that combine complex carbohydrates, protein, and fats to balance blood sugar levels.

Get plenty of omega-3 essential fatty acids, vitamins A, B, C, and E, and magnesium, zinc, and calcium. Consider supplementing with evening primrose oil and fish or krill oil. Try a whole-foods nutritional cleanse to support your liver.

Herbs such as dandelion and milk thistle strengthen the liver. Ginseng, black cohosh, and wild yam can often be effective in increasing sexual desire in women. Wild yam cream can replenish vaginal tissue to make sex more enjoyable. If you have your uterus or ovaries removed, see the suggestions in the menopausal chapter for herbs that help enhance hormonal balance.

Movement and Bodywork

To strengthen and heal your body in your effort to avoid hysterectomy, follow the movement guidelines in chapter five and the chapter in part three that pertains to your condition. Place a strong emphasis on activities that strengthen your core, improve posture, and decrease pain caused by compression—activities like those found in Pilates or yoga. It may be useful to work with a physical therapist or mind-body practitioner such as a chiropractor, energy healer, acupuncturist, or massage therapist, or a Feldenkrais or Alexander Technique teacher, to correct nerve tissue damage and develop new ways of movement that free up your body.

If you are going to have a hysterectomy, strengthen your core regularly to improve posture both before surgery and after recovery, to prevent common post-hysterectomy complications such as pelvic pain, incontinence, and compromised posture. The better your physical shape before surgery, the more quickly you can recover—so exercise as frequently as possible and include strength and interval training in your workout. If you are in too much pain or too exhausted before your surgery to perform vigorous exercise, use mild movement techniques such as Rosen Method Movement, tai chi, qi gong, and water exercise combined with daily stretching to gently strengthen your body, improve flexibility, and increase energy levels. Do Kegel exercises before surgery and for the rest of your life to strengthen your pelvic floor, improve sex, and prevent pelvic prolapse.

The type of hysterectomy you have will determine how long you need to wait before beginning abdominal exercises and aerobic activities other than walking in the hospital, at your home, or on other flat surfaces if approved by your surgeon. Follow your doctor's instructions about when it is safe to resume aerobic exercise, core strengthening, and any form of heavy lifting. Slowly transition back into your exercise routine, starting at a much easier level, and build back up over several weeks to reach your presurgery fitness levels.

After your complete recovery, use myofascial exercise systems such as the MELT Method or Yamuna Body Rolling to heal scar tissue, rehydrate myofascial connective tissue, and align your structure. Continue to do activities that help you strengthen your core, lengthen your spine, and develop healthy posture. Each week, pursue a variety of exercise options, including cardio activities with interval training, core stability, flexibility and balance, and strength training. Find activities you love or people you enjoy seeing during your workout to help make regular exercise a fun lifelong habit.

In several major hospitals across the United States, acupuncture is used right before and during surgery to improve outcomes and speed recovery. People who use acupuncture during surgery have less pain, use less pain medication, and have fewer side effects from medication during recovery. See whether there is a hospital in your area that offers acupuncture with your surgery or during recovery. If not, consider having acupuncture treatments before and after surgery to strengthen outcomes, decrease pain, and heal more quickly.

Conscious Breathing

Whether or not you choose to have a hysterectomy, deep breathing can help you reduce pain and restore your health. Using the instructions for conscious breathing in chapter three, find someplace you can relax and close your eyes. Begin to breathe long deep breaths in and out through your mouth. Imagine that every breath is helping you release pain and bring more vitality into your life.

With each inhalation, feel yourself receiving the energy of aliveness; with each exhalation, let go of pain and constriction. Imagine that powerful healing energy is flowing into your uterus and pelvic core with every breath. Sense that layers of stuck, congested energy are flowing out of your uterus and the surrounding area with every exhalation.

If you do not want to have a hysterectomy, use this breathing exercise for five to ten minutes each day in addition to the suggested breathwork in the chapter related to your uterine imbalance. Breathe in restoration and success. Sense that your uterus is already healed and that you are totally well.

If you choose to have a hysterectomy, use breathing before and after surgery to relax your body and breathe out pain. Each day during your entire recovery period, breathe in healing light, restorative energy, and vitality and breathe out pain or loss. When you feel your recovery is complete, breathe in creativity, sexuality, personal power, and feminine energy to the area of your body where your uterus was for five to ten minutes every day for the next several months.

Cognitive Restructuring

Cecelia was a forty-four-year-old family practice physician who had a hysterectomy the year before we spoke. Cecelia had undergone a myomectomy for uterine fibroids a few years before but then developed more fibroids. However, her menses had become so heavy that she had to curtail most of her non–work-related activities during her period, which could last as long as eight to ten days every month. Cecelia told me that she had wanted to keep her uterus for health reasons, but she felt that for her own sanity and the sake of her family, she could not go on living the way she was. She shared with me how she had finally decided to have a hysterectomy.

One day after a yoga class, Cecelia's instructor approached her and asked whether there was a reason she had been absent from class the last two weeks. When she told her about her problem, her yoga teacher mentioned that perhaps Cecelia could perform a ritual saying goodbye to her uterus. She had never thought about doing anything like that before, but her instructor mentioned that doing such a ritual might help her come to peace with the choice to have surgery and gain some closure on this part of her life.

Cecelia told me that she sat with this idea for a month. Even though she considered herself religious and somewhat spiritual, she had not been accustomed to planning rituals or spending much time contemplating something that was so interior. Eventually, Cecelia decided to take an afternoon off work and go to a large park in a nearby town so she would be sure not to see anyone she knew. She sat by a tree overlooking a valley, and when she was confident that nobody was around to possibly hear her, she started speaking to her uterus.

At first she felt awkward and very self-conscious, but after a few minutes she grew accustomed to it and felt as if, in taking this quiet time to speak to her body, she was greeting an old friend after many years of distance. Cecelia recalled that she told her uterus she appreciated all it had done for her. She was glad it was able to function for as long as it did and that she was able to bring her babies into the world with it. She then asked for forgiveness for all the years of cursing it for having her periods. She realized that before the fibroids had come along, her periods had not really been so bad after all. Then Cecelia asked for permission to remove her uterus. At that moment she felt great relief in her body, and she knew that a hysterectomy would be the right choice for her. For the first time in a long while, Cecelia felt at peace with herself and knew the surgery would help her heal.

Like Cecelia, you may find it helpful to journal, visualize, or talk to your body about the best course of action for you to take regarding your uterine health. Journal or ask your body whether there are other less-invasive surgical options, self-care practices, or mind-body treatments that would be helpful for you to try before having your uterus removed. Explore whether you hold any beliefs that prevent you from nourishing your health or being able to experience profound healing through more gentle means. If hysterectomy does seem like the right choice for you, journal on how you can support your health, creativity, sexuality, and feminine energy after the removal of your uterus.

Use stream-of-consciousness writing to journal about how your future will unfold if you do have a hysterectomy or if you choose not to. Let your subconscious wisdom flow onto the pages as you write about how you will feel, look, and be if you choose other health care options to address the uterine problems you are currently facing or if you decide to have a hysterectomy. Try to let go of all judgments and preconceived notions from yourself, your family, or your care providers as you connect with your inner knowing and write about the different ways your various treatment options will affect your future. It may also be helpful to do this same exercise using visualization.

Visualization

If you would prefer to not have a hysterectomy, employ guided imagery to imagine that the steps and treatments you do take to heal yourself will work perfectly. Visualize your health improving, your uterus becoming stronger, and your energy levels rejuvenating over the coming weeks and months. Picture that you quickly and easily find the right healers and doctors who assist you in resolving your uterine issues in a way that feels right to you. Connect with a future full of health, wellness, fun, and fulfillment. See yourself already healed every day. Use the imagery from chapter three and any chapter that pertains to your uterine condition daily to support your body as it heals.

If you are going to have a hysterectomy, visualize the procedure significantly improving your health. Envision your surgery team perfectly performing the hysterectomy. Imagine feeling better than expected in the hospital and during your recovery period at home. Picture yourself getting plenty of rest and easily receiving help from others who want to support you while you recover.

Sense that after your recovery you have more energy than before. Connect with this feeling of a bright new beginning and imagine all the fun you will have as you enjoy health in your life. See yourself eating and exercising in ways that truly enhance your health. Know that you made the right choice for you and that you can have abundant wellness for the rest of your life. Imagine your posture improving and your strength, passion, and energy levels expanding every year of your life.

If you do have a hysterectomy, use the visualizations in the previous chapter to support your endocrine system and help balance your hormones.

Belief Transformation Visualization and Ritual: This guided imagery describes a process of using elements such as fire or water to purify energy, emotions, beliefs, contracts, or agreements. I learned this ritual many years ago while studying traditional rites for cleansing and healing. Clients have enjoyed using this technique both as imagery and as ritual. Either way, it is an incredibly powerful process to release nonnourishing beliefs, agreements, and contracts and their associated emotions and feelings from your body and mind.

Before you begin this visualization, consider a belief, agreement, or contract you would like to release from your life. You may want to use the tools in the cognitive structuring sections of the book to help you identify any beliefs or unconscious contracts you may hold that no longer support you. Your belief might be about potential surgery or your uterine health, identity as a woman, personal power, or life purpose. If you are not sure which beliefs you would like to transform, go ahead and do the visualization and trust what comes up for you during this exercise.

To begin this imagery, follow the guidelines in chapter three. Allow yourself to breathe in and out of your mouth in a comfortable way. Become aware of your breath and relax your body. Envision yourself in a beautiful place in nature that has either a stream of water running through it or an outdoor fire in a fireplace or pit. This can be somewhere that you have seen or been to before or a place in your imagination.

Imagine that it is your favorite time of day and the perfect temperature for you. Know that you are totally safe. If you choose the water imagery, you may picture a flowing spring of blue water, a small meandering creek, or a large, quickly moving river. If you prefer fire, you may observe a roaring blaze in an outdoor fireplace made of bricks or embers burning brightly in a circular pit surrounded by smooth stones. You might also see a comfortable chaise or bench near the water or fire.

Envision that you can feel the fresh air on your skin, touch the soft earth underneath you, and hear either the water moving gently or the fire crackling nearby. Envision moving closer to the stream of water or the fire. Let yourself feel the freshness of the water or the warmth of the fire.

You may notice that there are containers or boxes near you. Know that each container holds sets of beliefs that you hold about yourself, others you know, or the world in general, or agreements that you have unconsciously made with others. Look at the containers and the labels on the outside of them. Open the containers and look through them, examining their contents.

Observe whether there are any beliefs, agreements, or contracts from the containers you would like to let go of, or whether there are any whole containers that you would now like to release. Take any sheets of paper or entire containers to the water or fire with you. If you do not picture any containers, simply imagine finding a pen and paper on a table next to the chair. Write down the belief, contract, or agreement you would now like to release.

Either stand or sit near the stream or fire and declare to yourself and the universe that you now release the beliefs, contracts, and their associated feelings and energies that you have felt in your body. Fully feel all of the energy and beliefs surfacing in your body as you begin to release the contracts or beliefs fully into the water or fire to be purified. Trust the power of your intent as you concentrate fully on letting go with every cell of your being.

After you have fully released all the agreements and energy that no longer serve you, envision that there is an easel nearby where you can write your new beliefs. Go to the desk and find paints, brushes, crayons, colored pencils, or a feathered quill pen and a large roll of paper, like an ancient scroll, on the desk. Imagine unrolling the scroll and cutting a swath of paper at least three feet wide. Use your utensil of choice and write your new empowering contracts, agreements, or beliefs on this paper.

Use as many large pieces from the scroll as you would like, inscribing each of the new beliefs, contracts, or agreements you want to establish in your consciousness on its own poster-sized piece of paper. See the tape on your desk and imagine that there is an outdoor wall nearby on which you can display all your new supportive agreements, beliefs, and contracts. As you look at your new agreements, let yourself feel all of the loving feelings connected to these contracts or beliefs fully in your body.

When you are through acknowledging yourself and the new energy you are creating in your life, express your gratitude and begin to leave your meditation, knowing you can come back as often as you would like to fill your being with more brilliance and light. Stretch your arms and legs and when you are ready to come back to the room, open your eyes, feeling revived and peaceful.

Turn this visualization into a ritual by writing down contracts that you no longer want, ripping up the paper, and burning it in any fire-safe container. Place the ashes in a river or some sort of moving body of water to further release them out of your life. Write new nourishing beliefs or agreements.

Trust Your Inner Wisdom

Only you can know what is best for your body. If you do decide to have a hysterectomy, consider doing some sort of ritual to honor your uterus and the sacredness of your body. This might be as simple as consciously saying goodbye to your uterus or a more elaborate process that calls in healing energy for your procedure and recovery. If you choose to heal your body while you keep your uterus, use the self-care practices in this book in combination with biomedical or mind-body treatments. Know that you can restore your health through a variety of methods. Whatever decision you make, caring for yourself with whole-foods nutrition, regular exercise, deep breathing, cognitive restructuring, and visualization will help you create lifelong wellness.

Creating Lifelong Wellness: New Possibilities for Uterine Health

During my medical anthropology research in the United States, I noticed that most women with persistent menopausal symptoms had experienced problems with menstruation and other uterine disorders earlier in their lives. This pattern seemed significant to me, but when I mentioned it to gynecologists in my research they were rarely intrigued by my observation. I realized that instead of looking at women's lifelong uterine health, conventional medical ideology encourages physicians to view menstruation, fertility, pregnancy, and menopause as separate areas of focus. Consequently, problems that arise during these stages are generally treated as distinct and unrelated to uterine conditions that occurred earlier in life and are seldom thought to increase risks for future uterine difficulties—even though research shows an association between PMS, menstrual irregularities, menopausal symptoms, and osteoporosis.[1]

As I have illustrated, benign uterine health problems are your body's way of telling you there are underlying imbalances that need to be corrected. If you experience uterine difficulties and take actions that only relieve the symptoms without addressing the root causes, you are more likely to experience additional uterine problems and other health concerns later in life. Menstruation, fertility, pregnancy, and menopause are intricately connected to your uterine, endocrine, hormonal, and digestive health. Many researchers consider PMS a mineral deficiency condition, brought on by calcium or magnesium deficiency. If actions are not taken to improve nutrition and slow nutrient loss, these mineral deficiencies can continue to create hormonal imbalances that make conception and menopause more difficult, may cause other benign uterine disease, and certainly increase the risk of osteoporosis. Fortunately, the mind-body practices in this book provide healthy, sustainable solutions you can use to help heal uterine imbalances and create lifelong wellness. If you begin to take care of your uterus now, it will be around later to help take care of you.

The Benefits of Prevention

We now know that the uterus contributes to women's whole body health in many important ways. It is essential that we share this knowledge through public outreach to ensure that all women learn that it is vital to care for the uterus as part of overall wellness. We are all familiar with the benefits of using exercise, nutrition, and stress reduction to help prevent high blood pressure, heart disease, diabetes, and osteoporosis. We can also apply a similar approach to support our uteruses and reduce our high rates of hysterectomy and benign uterine disease. It is my hope that this message of prevention will become an integral part of patient education, enabling more women to enjoy the many benefits the uterus provides. This public outreach needs to be specifically targeted to teenage women and girls. If young women understand the importance of supporting the uterus through healthy lifestyles, future generations will be able to significantly lower their incidence of benign uterine disease and cultivate lifelong wellness.

I believe that gynecologists have not emphasized nutritional and lifestyle prevention strategies for uterine health as much as some other medical fields because biomedicine historically considered the uterus as naturally problematic and dispensable. People in Western society have been socialized to view benign uterine problems as normal and unavoidable. Our expectations of difficulties with menstruation and menopause have been shaped by our cultural tendency to stigmatize female bodily processes that may inconvenience men or lower our productivity. We rarely hear physicians suggest that men remove their reproductive organs. However, in the United States some doctors regularly tell women that the uterus (and ovaries) are disposable.

Yet recent research shows that, like the ovaries, the uterus is vitally important beyond reproduction. The uterus contributes to your physical, emotional, and sexual health in many essential ways. It produces chemicals that help lower your blood pressure and reduce your risk of heart disease. The uterus enhances your posture and can increase your sexual pleasure.

We now know that women in some non-Western societies do not have such high rates of benign uterine disorders as women in the West do. Along with having different reproductive, nutrition, and lifestyle patterns, these cultures frequently consider menstruation and menopause as positive processes. I believe this is because many of these societies have religious beliefs that revere the divine feminine as well as the divine masculine and recognize all life-forms as valuable. Thus, people in these societies are raised to view female bodies as well as male bodies as sacred. Learning about these cultures and their beliefs can offer us powerful insights for understanding uterine health as well as the holistic nature of life.

Early humans were so in awe of the transformative and creative power of the uterus that they painted it on cave walls. I encourage you to release any stigma you have learned about the uterus and create your own rituals to celebrate and nourish your body. Find authentic ways you can honor your body and uterine processes. Profound healing will happen more easily if you discard any cultural attitudes that do not acknowledge your inherent infinite self-worth. If you simply shift from using biomedical to mind-body treatments without transforming your beliefs, you may not obtain the results you desire. Along with incorporating nutrition, exercise, and stress reduction into your life, develop beliefs that affirm your right to be healthy and happy.

Expanding Uterine Power

On an energetic level, your uterus has several potent meanings. The uterus is a vessel for creativity, transformation, and relationships. Engaging in creative pursuits of all kinds can help strengthen your uterine health. Make plenty of time in your life for dance, art, writing, painting, gardening, or any other kind of creativity that you enjoy. Start to look for ways you can express your creativity in every area of your life and work.

Feed your uterine health by building satisfying relationships in your life. Explore what it is like to express yourself freely during your interactions with others. If you have some relationships in your life that do not satisfy you or leave you feeling inadequate, spend less time with those people and instead focus more on connections with people you enjoy. Including more health-conscious people in your social network will help enhance your own wellness. Creating harmony in your relationships will give you more energy to take care of yourself.

Always make plenty of time for your most important relationship—the one with yourself. As women we are constantly giving of ourselves to others. However, at its very essence, feminine energy is about receiving. It is important to establish traditions that help you nurture your own energy on a daily basis. Discover how you can receive as much nourishment as possible in your life and release all habits that involve taking in debilitating energy from others.

Meditate, breathe, visualize, or do other practices that help you rejuvenate regularly. Use the exercises in the book to strengthen your awareness of energy in your life. Use visualization to amplify and expand the energies you want in your life such as health and joy while decreasing the qualities you want less of such as disease and fatigue. Cultivate vitality in all your interactions and enjoy life to the fullest.

Holistic healing traditions offer beneficial new ways of viewing your health. Everything in your mind, body, and spirit is connected. It is important to care for your uterus and every other part of your being to foster wellness. Believe in your body's innate ability to heal, and provide it with the support it needs. Together, as women aligned in power and health, we can give birth to a world full of peace and freedom.

Resources

Cognitive Restructuring

Grason, Sandy. *Journalution: Journaling to Awaken Your Inner Voice, Heal Your Life, and Manifest Your Dreams.* Novato, CA: New World Library, 2005.

Hay, Louise. *Heal Your Body: The Mental Causes for Physical Illness and the Metaphysical Way to Overcome Them.* Carlsbad, CA: Hay House, Inc., 1984.

International Coach Federation-Life Coach Directory
www.coachfederation.org
International Coach Federation
2365 Harrodsburg Rd., Suite A325
Lexington, KY 40504
888-423-3131

Conscious Breathing

Kizer, Ken, and Kizer, Renee. *Path to Freedom: Using Conscious Connected Breathing and Astrology for Emotional Healing.* Richmond, VA: Center for Awareness, 1991.

Manne, Joy. *Conscious Breathing: How Shamanic Breathing Can Change Your Life.* Berkeley, CA: North Atlantic Books, 2004.

Energy Healing and Bodywork Techniques

Blum, Jeanne Elizabeth. *Woman Heal Thyself: An Ancient Healing System for Contemporary Women*. North Clarendon, VT: Tuttle Publishing, 1996.

Byers, Dwight C. *Better Health with Foot Reflexology: The Original Ingham Method*. Saint Petersburg, FL: Ingham Publishing, 1983.

Craniosacral therapy
www.upledger.com
The Upledger Institute
11211 Prosperity Farms Rd., Suite D-325
Palm Beach Gardens, FL 33410
800-233-5880 or 561-622-4334

Emotional Freedom Technique—Acupressure tapping
www.emofree.com

International Association of Healthcare Practitioners—Mind-body practitioner
directory
www.iahp.com

Network chiropractic
www.associationfornetworkcare.com
Association for Network Care
444 West Main Street
Longmont, CA 80501
303-678-8101

Reiki practitioners and products
www.reikialliance.com
Reiki Alliance
204 N. Chestnut Street
Kellogg, ID 83837
208-783-3535

Mind-Body Movement and Postural Alignment Techniques

Alexander Technique classes and DVDs
www.alexandertech.org
American Society for the Alexander Technique
PO Box 60008
Florence, MA 01062
800-473-0620

Feldenkrais Method classes and resources
www.feldenkrais.com
The Feldenkrais Method of Somatic Education
5436 N. Albina Ave
Portland, OR 97217
800-775-2118 or 503-221-6612

MELT Method classes and resources
www.meltmethod.com

Nia Technique classes and DVDs
www.nianow.com
Nia International Headquarters
918 SW Yamhill, 3rd Floor
Portland, OR 97205
503-245-9886

Rosen Method Movement classes and DVDs
www.rosenmethod.org
Rosen Method Center
825 Bancroft Way
Berkeley, CA 94710
510-845-6606

Yamuna Body Rolling classes and DVDs
www.yamunabodyrolling.com

Natural Birthing

England, Pam, and Holowitz, Rob. *Birthing from Within: An Extra-Ordinary Guide to Childbirth Preparation.* Albuquerque, NM: Partera Press, 1998.

Gaskin, Ina Mae. *Ina May's Guide to Childbirth.* New York: Bantam Books, 2003.

Mongan, Marie F. *Hypnobirthing: A Celebration of Life.* Concord, NH: Rivertree Publishing, 1998.

Scott, Pauline. *Sit Up and Take Notice: Positioning Yourself for a Better Birth.* Taranga, New Zealand: Great Scott Publications, 2003.

Nutrition

Ellis, Lesley. *Seven Day Detox Plan: Change Your Eating Habits for Life.* New York: Foulsham, 2000.

L'Esperance, Carrie. *The Seasonal Detox Diet: Remedies from the Ancient Cookfire.* Rochester, VT: Healing Arts Press, 2002.

Pollan, Michael. *The Omnivore's Dilemma: A Natural History of Four Meals.* New York: Penguin Books, 2006.

Visualization

Gawain, Shakti. *Creative Visualization: Use the Power of Your Imagination to Create What You Want in Your Life.* San Rafael, CA: New World Library, 1995.

Naparstek, Belleruth. *Staying Well with Guided Imagery.* New York: Warner Books, 1994.

Rossman, Martin. *Guided Imagery for Self-Healing: An Essential Resource for Anyone Seeking Wellness.* Novato, CA: New World Library, 2000.

Notes

Introduction

1. All names in the book have been changed to honor the privacy of research subjects.
2. Margaret Lock, "The Politics of Mid-Life and Menopause: Ideologies for the Second Sex in North America and Japan," in *Knowledge, Power, and Practice: The Anthropology of Medicine in Everyday Life*, eds. Shirley Lindenbaum and Margaret Lock (Berkeley: University of California Press, 1993), 330–363.
3. J. K. Ockene, et al., "Symptom Experience After Discontinuing Use of Estrogen Plus Progestin," *Journal of the American Medical Association* 294 (2) (July 2005): 183–193.

Chapter One

1. Michio Kaku, *Visions: How Science Will Revolutionize the Twenty-First Century* (New York: Doubleday, 1997), 196.
2. Emily Martin, *The Woman in the Body: A Cultural Analysis of Reproduction* (Boston, MA: Beacon Press, 1987).

Chapter Two

1. Deborah Sundahl, *Female Ejaculation and the G-Spot: Not Your Mother's Orgasm Book* (Alameda, CA: Hunter House, 2003), 47.
2. Christa Schulte, *Tantric Sex for Women: A Guide for Lesbian, Bi, Hetero, and Solo Lovers* (Berlin: Krug and Schadenberg, 2005), 201.

3. Susan Love, *Dr. Susan Love's Hormone Book: Making Informed Choices About Menopause* (New York: Random House, 1997), 177.

4. Margie Profit, "Menstruation as a Defense Against Pathogens Transported by Sperm," *Quarterly Review of Biology*, 68 (3) (Sept 1993): 335–381.

5. J. D. Shelton, "Prostacyclin from the Uterus and Woman's Cardiovascular Advantage," *Prostaglandins Leukotrienes and Medicine*, 8 (5) (May 1982): 459–466.

6. Natalie Angier, *Woman: An Intimate Geography* (New York: Anchor Books, 2000), 121.

7. Jane Ballantyne and Jianren Mao, "Opioid Therapy for Chronic Pain," *New England Journal of Medicine*, 349 (Nov 2003): 1943–1953.

8. A. S. Taylor, C. Ang, S. C. Bell, and J. C. Konje, "The Role of the Endocannabinoid System in Gametogenesis, Implantation, and Early Pregnancy," *Human Reproduction Update* 13 (5) (June 2007): 501–513.

Chapter Three

1. J. Dvivedi et al., "Effect of '61-Points Relaxation Technique' on Stress Parameters in Premenstrual Syndrome," *Indian Journal of Physiology and Pharmacology* 52 (1) (Jan–Mar 2008): 69–76.

2. S. T. Sigmon and R. O. Nelson, "The Effectiveness of Activity Scheduling and Relaxation Training in the Treatment of Spasmodic Dysmenorrhea," *Journal of Behavioral Medicine* 11 (5) (Oct 1988): 483–495.

3. E. Zaborowska et al., "Effects of Acupuncture, Applied Relaxation, Estrogens, and Placebo on Hot Flushes in Postmenopausal Women: An Analysis of Two Prospective, Parallel, Randomized Studies," *Climacteric* 10 (1) (June 2007): 38–45.

4. Herbert Benson and Marg Stark, *Timeless Healing: The Power and Biology of Belief* (New York: Scribner, 1996), 147.

5. R. R. Freedman and S. Woodward, "Behavioral Treatment of Menopausal Hot Flushes: Evaluation by Ambulatory Monitoring," *American Journal of Obstetrics and Gynecology* 167 (2) (1992): 436–439.

6. I. L. Goodale, A. D. Domar, and H. Benson, "Alleviation of Premenstrual Syndrome Symptoms with the Relaxation Response," *Obstetrics and Gynecology* 75 (4) (1990): 649–655.

7. M. Groer and C. Ohnesorge, "Menstrual-Cycle Lengthening and Reduction in Premenstrual Distress Through Guided Imagery," *Journal of Holistic Nursing* 11 (3) (1993): 286–294.

8. Barbara Rees, "Effect of Relaxation with Guided Imagery on Anxiety, Depression, and Self-Esteem in Primiparas," *Journal of Holistic Nursing* 13 (3) (1995): 255–267.

9. C. H. McKinney et al., "Effects of Guided Imagery and Music (GIM) Therapy on Mood and Cortisol in Healthy Adults," *Health Psychology* (4) (July 1997): 390–400.

10. C. A. Morse et al., "A Comparison of Hormone Therapy, Coping Skills Training, and Relaxation for the Relief of Premenstrual Syndrome," *Journal of Behavioral Medicine* 14 (5) (1991): 469–489.

11. L. Keefer and E. B. Blanchard, "A Behavioral Group Treatment Program for Menopausal Hot Flashes: Results of a Pilot Study," *Applied Psychophysiology and Biofeedback* 30 (1) (Mar 2005): 21–30.

12. Lazaris, *Forgiveness: The Miracle of Magic* (Raleigh, NC: NPN Publishing, Inc., 2004), audiocassette.

13. Don Miguel Ruiz, *The Four Agreements: A Practical Guide to Personal Freedom* (San Rafael, CA: Amber-Allen Publishing, 1997), 4.

Chapter Four

1. N. D. Barnard et al., "Diet and Sex-Hormone Binding Globulin, Dysmenorrheal, and Premenstrual Symptoms," *Obstetrics and Gynecology* (2) (Feb 2000): 245–250.

2. F. Parazzini et al., "Selected Food Intake and Risk of Endometriosis," *Human Reproduction* 19 (8) (July 2004): 1755–1759.

3. P. Albertazzi et al., "The Effect of Dietary Soy Supplementation on Hot Flashes," *Obstetrics and Gynecology* 91 (1) (1998): 6–11.

4. T. Fujiwara, "Skipping Breakfast Is Associated with Dysmenorrhea in Young Women in Japan," *International Journal of Food Science Nutrition* 54 (6) (Nov 2003): 505–509.

5. J. R. Mathias et al., "Relation of Endometriosis and Neuromuscular Disease of the Gastrointestinal Tract: New Insights," *Fertility and Sterility* 70 (1) (July 1998): 81–88.

6. Dian Sheppardson Mills and Michael Vernon, *Endometriosis: A Key to Healing Through Nutrition* (London: Thorsons; New York: Harper Collins, 1999), 278.

7. S. Gallager, "Omega 3 Oils and Pregnancy," *Midwifery Today with International Midwife* 69 (Spring 2004): 26–31.

8. B. J. Abelow, T. R. Holford, and K. L. Insogna, "Cross-Cultural Association Between Dietary Animal Protein and Hip Fracture: A Hypothesis," *Calcified Tissue International* 50 (1) (Jan 1992): 14–18.

9. Christiane Northrup, *Women's Bodies, Women's Wisdom: Creating Physical and Emotional Health and Healing* (New York: Bantam Books, 2006), 577.

10. Donna Thorpe et al., "Effects of Meat Consumption and Vegetarian Diet on Risk of Wrist Fracture over 25 Years in a Cohort of Peri- and Postmenopausal Women," *Public Health Nutrition* 11 (2008): 564–572.

Chapter Five

1. S. J. Britnell et al., "Postural Health in Women: The Role of Physiotherapy," *Journal of Obstetrics and Gynaecology Canada* (159) (May 2005): 493–500.

2. J. F. Steege and J. A. Blumenthal, "The Effects of Aerobic Exercise on Premenstrual Symptoms in Middle-Aged Women: A Preliminary Study," *Journal of Psychosomatic Research* 37 (2) (1993): 127–133.

3. N. Teoman, A. Ozcan, and B. Acar, "The Effect of Exercise on Physical Fitness and Quality of Life in Postmenopausal Women," *Maturitas* 47 (1) (Jan 2004): 71–77.

4. Elaine Meadows, "Treatments for Patients with Pelvic Pain," *Urologic Nursing* 19 (1) (March 1999): 33–35.

5. Maxwell Walsh and Barbara Polus, "A Randomized, Placebo-Controlled Clinical Trial on the Efficacy of Chiropractic Therapy on Premenstrual Syndrome," *Journal of Manipulative and Physiological Therapeutics* 22 (9) (Nov–Dec 1999): 582–585.

6. L. J. Wurn et al., "Treating Endometriosis Pain with a Manual Pelvic Physical Therapy," *Fertility and Sterility* 86 (3) (Sept 2006): S29–S30.

Chapter Six

1. Elizabeth R. Bertone-Johnson et al., "Calcium and Vitamin D Intake and Risk of Incident Premenstrual Syndrome," *Archives of Internal Medicine* 165 (11) (June 2005): 1246–1252.

2. Tori Hudson, *Women's Encyclopedia of Natural Medicine: Alternative Therapies and Integrative Medicine for Total Health and Wellness* (New York: McGraw Hill, 2008), 10–11.

3. J. A. Aganoff and G. J. Boyle, "Aerobic Exercise, Mood States, and Menstrual Cycle Symptoms," *Journal of Psychosomatic Research* 38 (3) (1994): 183–192.

4. C. A. Morse et al., "A Comparison of Hormone Therapy, Coping Skills Training, and Relaxation for the Relief of Premenstrual Syndrome," *Journal of Behavioral Medicine* 14 (5) (1991): 469–489.

Chapter Seven

1. I. A. Bergqvist, L. Hummelshoj, G. Haegerstam, et al., "Enhancing Quality of Life in Women and Girls with Endometriosis-Related Pain When Traditional Treatments Have Failed," *Savonlinna* (July 2000): 11–12.

2. Parazzini, "Selected Food Intake," (see chap. 4, n. 2).

3. S. E. Rier, D. C. Martin, R. E. Bowman, et al., "Endometriosis in Rhesus Monkeys (*Maccaca mulatta*) Following Chronic Exposure to 2,3, 7,8-Tetra-chlorodibenzo-p-dioxin," *Fundamental and Applied Toxicology* 21 (1993): 433–441.

4. Martin Rossman, *Guided Imagery for Self-Healing: An Essential Resource for Anyone Seeking Wellness* (Novato, CA: New World Library, 2000), 72.

Chapter Eight

1. Lilian Thompson. "Dietary Flaxseed Alters Tumor Biological Markers in Postmenopausal Breast Cancer," *Clinical Cancer Research* 11 (May 2005): 3828–3835.

2. K. Sahin et al., "Lycopene Supplementation Prevents the Development of Spontaneous Smooth Muscle Tumors on the Oviduct in Japanese Quail," *Nutrition and Cancer* 50 (2) (2004): 181–189.

3. Northrup, *Women's Bodies, Women's Wisdom* (see chap. 4, n. 9).

Chapter Nine

1. Stacy Foren, James Flood, et al., "Measurement of Mercury Levels in Concentrated Over-the-Counter Fish Oil Preparations: Is Fish Oil Healthier Than Fish?" *Archives of Pathology and Laboratory Medicine* 127 (12) (July 2003): 1603–1605.

2. Edoardo Rossi, "Fish Oil Derivatives As a Prophylaxis of Recurrent Miscarriage Associated with Antiphospholipid Antibodies (APL): A Pilot Study," *Lupus* 2 (5) (1993): 319–323.

3. B. F. Wurn et al., "Treating Female Infertility and Improving IVF Pregnancy Rates with a Manual Physical Therapy Technique," *Medscape General Medicine* 6 (2) (June 2004): 51.

4. Kjell Salvesen and Siv Morkved, "Randomised Controlled Trial of Pelvic Floor Muscle Training During Pregnancy," *British Journal of Medicine* (329) (July 2004): 378–80.

5. Pauline Scott, *Sit Up and Take Notice: Positioning Yourself for a Better Birth* (Tauranga, New Zealand: Great Scott Publications, 2003), 104.

Chapter Ten

1. Bahram H. Arjmandi, Dania A. Khalil, Brenda J. Smith, et al., "Soy Protein Has a Greater Effect on Bone in Postmenopausal Women Not on Hormone Replacement Therapy, As Evidenced by Reducing Bone Resorption and Urinary Calcium Excretion," *The Journal of Clinical Endocrinology & Metabolism* 88 (3) (2003): 1048–1054.

2. Mary Taylor et al., "Participant Perspective on a Yoga Intervention for Menopausal Symptoms," *Complementary Health Practice Review* 13 (3) (2008): 171–181.

3. J. Williamson, A. White, A. Hart, and E. Ernst, "Randomised Controlled Trial of Reflexology for Menopausal Symptoms," *BJOG: An International Journal of Obstetrics and Gynaecology* 109 (9) (Sept. 2002): 1050–1055.

Chapter Eleven

1. Steven J. Bernstein, David E. Kanouse, and Brian S. Mitman, *Hysterectomy: Clinical Recommendations and Indications for Use* (Santa Monica, CA: Rand, 1997), 42.

2. William H. Parker, Michael S. Broder, Zhimei Liu, Donna Shoupe, et al., "Ovarian Conservation at the Time of Hysterectomy for Benign Disease," *Obstetrics and Gynecology*, 106 (2) (August 2005): 219–226.

Conclusion

1. S. J. Lee and J. A. Kanis, "An Association Between Osteoporosis and Premenstrual Symptoms and Postmenopausal Symptoms," *Bone and Mineral* 24 (2) (Feb 1994): 127–134.

Bibliography

Abelow, B. J., Holford, T. R., and Insogna, K. L. "Cross-Cultural Association Between Dietary Animal Protein and Hip Fracture: A Hypothesis." *Calcified Tissue International* 50 (1) (January 1992): 14–18.

Aganoff, J. A., and Boyle, G. J. "Aerobic Exercise, Mood States and Menstrual Cycle Symptoms." *Journal Psychosomatic Research* 38 (3) (1994): 183–192.

Albertazzi, P., et al. "The Effect of Dietary Soy Supplementation on Hot Flashes." *Obstetrics and Gynecology* 91 (1) (1998): 6–11.

Amadiume, Ife. *Male Daughters, Female Husbands.* London: Zed Books, 1987.

Anderson, D., et al. "Menopause in Australia and Japan: Effects of Country of Residence on Menopausal Status and Menopausal Symptoms." *Climacteric* 7 (2) (June 2004): 165–174.

Anderson, David E., McNeely, Jessica D., Chesney, Margaret A., and Windham, Beverly G. "Breathing Variability at Rest Is Positively Associated with 24-h Blood Pressure Level." *American Journal of Hypertension* (25) (September 2008): 1324–1329.

Angier, Natalie. *Woman: An Intimate Geography.* New York: Anchor Books, 2000.

Arjmandi, Bahram H., Khalil, Dania A., Smith, Brenda J., et al. "Soy Protein Has a Greater Effect on Bone in Postmenopausal Women Not on Hormone Replacement Therapy, As Evidenced by Reducing Bone Resorption and Urinary Calcium Excretion." *The Journal of Clinical Endocrinology & Metabolism* 88 (3) (2003): 1048–1054.

Avis, Nancy E., and Crawford, Sybil. "Cultural Differences in Symptoms and Attitudes Toward Menopause." *Menopause Management* 17 (3) (May/June 2008): 8–13.

Ballantyne, Jane, and Mao, Jianren. "Opiod Therapy for Chronic Pain." *New England Journal of Medicine* 349 (Nov 2003): 1943–1953.

Barnard, N. D., et al. "Diet and Sex-Hormone Binding Globulin, Dysmenorrheal, and Premenstrual Symptoms." *Obstetrics & Gynecology* (2) (Feb. 2000): 245–250.

Barton, D. L., et al. "Prospective Evaluation of Vitamin E for Hot Flashes in Breast Cancer Survivors." *Journal of Clinical Oncology* 16 (1998): 495–500.

Bazzo, Debbie, and Moeller, Ruth Ann. "Imagine This! Infinite Uses of Guided Imagery in Women's Health." *Journal of Holistic Nursing* 17 (4) (1999): 317–330.

Beck, Peggy V., Walters, Anna Lee, and Francisco, Nia. *The Sacred: Ways of Knowledge, Sources of Life*. Tsaile, AZ: Navajo Community College Press, 1977.

Benson, Herbert, and Stark, Marg. *Timeless Healing: The Power and Biology of Belief*. New York: Scribner, 1996.

Berger, Gabriella, and Wenzel, Eberhard. "Women, Body and Society: Cross-cultural Differences in Menopause Experiences." *Public Health Virtual Library*, September 2001.

Bergqvist, I. A., et al. "Enhancing Quality of Life in Women and Girls with Endometriosis-Related Pain When Traditional Treatments Have Failed." *Savonlinna* (July 2000): 11–12.

Bernstein, Steven J., Kanouse, David E., and Mitman, Brian S. *Hysterectomy: Clinical Recommendations and Indications for Use*. Santa Monica, CA: Rand, 1997.

Bertone-Johnson, Elizabeth R., et al. "Calcium and Vitamin D Intake and Risk of Incident Premenstrual Syndrome." *Archives of Internal Medicine* 165 (11) (June 2005): 1246–1252.

Beyene, Yewoubdar. *From Menarche to Menopause: Reproductive Lives of Peasant Women in Two Cultures*. Albany, NY: State University of New York Press, 1989.

Beyene, Yewoubdar, and Martin, Mary C. "Menopausal Experiences and Bone Density of Mayan Women in Yucatan, Mexico." *American Journal of Human Biology* 13 (4) (May 2001): 505–511.

Blake, F., Salkovskis, P., et al. "Cognitive Therapy for Premenstrual Syndrome: A Controlled Trial." *Journal of Psychosomatic Research* 45 (4) (1998): 307–318.

Britnell, S. J., et al. "Postural Health in Women: The Role of Physiotherapy." *Journal of Obstetrics and Gynaecology Canada* (159) (May 2005): 493–500.

Brown, Joseph Epes. *The Sacred Pipe: Black Elk's Account of the Seven Rites of the Oglala Sioux*. Baltimore, MD: Penguin Books, 1971.

Buckley, Thomas, and Gottlieb, Alma, eds. *Blood Magic: The Anthropology of Menstruation*. Berkeley, CA: University of California Press, 1988.

Calais-Germain, Blandine. *Anatomy of Breathing*. Seattle, WA: Eastland Press, 2006.

Campbell, T. Colin, and Campbell, Thomas M. II. *The China Study: The Most Comprehensive Study of Nutrition Ever Conducted*. Dallas, TX: Benbella Books, 2005.

Chirawatkul, Siriporn, and Manderson, Lenore. "Perceptions of Menopause in Northeast Thailand: Contested Meaning and Practice." *Social Science & Medicine* 39 (11) (1994): 1545–1554.

Clifton, Lucille. *Blessing the Boats: New and Selected Poems 1988–2000*. Rochester, NY: BOA Editions, 2000.

Cohen, Ken. *The Way of Qigong: The Art and Science of Chinese Healing*. New York: Ballantine, 1997.

Connelly, Diane. *Traditional Acupuncture: The Law of the Five Elements*. Columbia, MD: Traditional Acupuncture Institute, 1994.

Davis, Dona. "The Meaning of Menopauses in a Newfoundland Fishing Village." *Culture, Medicine, and Psychiatry* 10 (March 1986): 73–94.

Davis-Floyd, Robbie. *Birth as an American Rite of Passage*. Berkeley, CA: University of California Press, 1992.

De Angelis, Lissa, and Siple, Molly. *SOS for PMS: Whole-Foods Solutions for Premenstrual Syndrome*. New York: Plume, 1999.

Delaney, J., Lupton, M. J., and Toth, E. *The Curse: A Cultural History of Menstruation*. Chicago, IL: University of Illinois Press, 1988.

Deutch, B. "Menstrual Discomfort in Danish Women Reduced by Dietary Supplements of Omega-3 PUFA and B_{12} (fish oil and seal oil capsules)." *Nutrition Research* 20 (5) (2000): 621–631.

Domar, Alice, and Dreher, Henry. *Healing Mind, Healthy Woman: Using the Mind-Body Connection to Manage Stress and Take Control of Your Life*. New York: Dell Publishing, 1996.

Dvivedi, J., et al. "Effect of '61-Points Relaxation Technique' on Stress Parameters in Premenstrual Syndrome." *Indian Journal of Physiology and Pharmacology* 52 (1) (2008): 69–76.

Eisler, Riane. *The Chalice and the Blade: Our History, Our Future*. San Francisco: CA: Harper Collins, 1995.

England, Pam, and Holowitz, Rob. *Birthing From Within: An Extra-Ordinary Guide to Childbirth Preparation*. Albuquerque, NM: Partera Press, 1998.

Flint, Marsha. "The Menopause: Reward or Punishment." *Psychosomatics* 16 (1975): 161–163.

Flint, Marsha, Kronengerg, Fredi, and Utian, Wolf, eds. *Multidisciplinary Perspectives on Menopause*. New York: New York Academy of Sciences, 1990.

Flint, Marsha, and Samil, Suprapti Ratua. "Cultural and Subcultural Meanings of Menopause." In *Multidisciplinary Perspectives on Menopause*, edited by Flint, Marsha, Kronengerg, Fredi, and Utian, Wolf. New York: New York Academy of Sciences, 1990, 134–148.

Foren, Stacy, Flood, James, et al. "Measurement of Mercury Levels in Concentrated Over-the-Counter Fish Oil Preparations: Is Fish Oil Healthier Than Fish?" *Archives of Pathology and Laboratory Medicine* 127 (12) (July 2003): 1603–1605.

Freedman, R. R., and Woodward, S. "Behavioral Treatment of Menopausal Hot Flushes: Evaluation by Ambulatory Monitoring." *American Journal of Obstetrics & Gynecology* 167 (2) (1992): 436–439.

Fujiwara, T. "Skipping Breakfast Is Associated with Dysmenorrhea in Young Women in Japan." *International Journal of Food Science Nutrition* 54 (6) (2003): 505–509.

Gallager, S. "Omega 3 Oils and Pregnancy." *Midwifery Today with International Midwife* 69 (Spring 2004): 26–31.

Gaskin, Ina Mae. *Ina May's Guide to Childbirth*. New York: Bantam Books, 2003.

Gawain, Shakti. *Creative Visualization: Use the Power of Your Imagination to Create What You Want in Your Life*. San Rafael, CA: New World Library, 1995.

Gerber, Richard. *Vibrational Medicine: The #1 Handbook of Subtle-Energy Therapies*. Rochester, VT: Bear & Company, 2001.

Gimputas, Marija. *The Language of the Goddess: Unearthing the Hidden Symbols of Western Civilization*. London: Thames and Hudson, 2001.

Gimputas, Marija. *The Living Goddesses*. Berkeley, CA: University of California Press, 1999.

Goodale, I. L., Domar, A. D., and Benson, H. "Alleviation of Premenstrual Syndrome Symptoms with the Relaxation Response." *Obstetrics and Gynecology* 75 (4) (1990): 649–655.

Goodwin, Scott C., and Broder, Michael. *What Your Doctor May Not Tell You About Fibroids: New Techniques and Therapies—Including Breakthrough Alternatives to Hysterectomy*. New York: Warner Books, 2003.

Grahn, Judy. *Blood, Bread, and Roses: How Menstruation Created the World*. Boston, MA: Beacon Press, 1994.

Grahn, Judy. "Goddess of the Blood Life Part One." *Metaformia: A Journal of Menstruation and Culture*, 2007.

Grason, Sandy. *Journalution: Journaling to Awaken Your Inner Voice, Heal Your Life, and Manifest Your Dreams*. Novato, CA: New World Library, 2005.

Groer, M., and Ohnesorge, C. "Menstrual-Cycle Lengthening and Reduction in Premenstrual Distress Through Guided Imagery." *Journal of Holistic Nursing* 11 (3) (1993): 286–294.

Haas, Adelaide, and Puretz, Susan L. *The Woman's Guide to Hysterectomy: Expectations and Options.* Berkeley, CA: Celestial Arts, 2002.

hooks, bell. *Feminist Theory, from Margin to Center.* Boston, MA: South End Press, 1984.

Hudson, Tori. *Women's Encyclopedia of Natural Medicine: Alternative Therapies and Integrative Medicine for Total Health and Wellness.* New York: McGraw Hill, 2008.

Jordan, Brigitte. *Birth in Four Cultures: A Crosscultural Investigation of Childbirth in Yucatan, Holland, Sweden, and the United States.* Prospect Heights, IL: Waveland Press, 1993.

Kaku, Michio. *Visions: How Science Will Revolutionize the Twenty-First Century.* New York: Doubleday, 1997.

Keefer, L., and Blanchard, E. B.. "A Behavioral Group Treatment Program for Menopausal Hot Flashes: Results of a Pilot Study." *Applied Psychophysiology and Biofeedback* 30 (1) (Mar 2005): 21–30.

Kizer, Ken, and Kizer, Renee. *Path to Freedom: Using Conscious Connected Breathing and Astrology for Emotional Healing.* Richmond, VA: Center for Awareness, 1991.

Knight, Chris. *Blood Relations: Menstruation and the Origins of Culture.* New Haven, CT: Yale University Press, 1991.

Lawlor, Robert. *Voices of the First Day: Awakening the Aboriginal Dreamtime.* Rochester, VT: Inner Traditions International, 1991.

Lee, John R., and Hopkins, Virginia. *What Your Doctor May Not Tell You About Menopause: The Breakthrough Book on Natural Hormone Balance.* New York: Wellness Central Hachette Book Group, 2004.

Lee, S. J., and Kanis, J. A. An Association Between Osteoporosis and Premenstrual Symptoms and Postmenopausal Symptoms." *Bone and Mineral* 24 (2) (Feb 1994): 127–134.

Lichtenstein, Alice, and Russell, Robert. "Essential Nutrients: Food or Supplements?" *Journal of the American Medical Association* 294 (3) (July 2005): 351–358.

Lincoln, Bruce. *Emerging from the Chrysalis: Rituals of Women's Initiation.* Cambridge, MA: Harvard University Press, 1981.

Lock, Margaret. "The Politics of Mid-Life and Menopause: Ideologies for the Second Sex in North America and Japan." In *Knowledge, Power, & Practice:*

The Anthropology of Medicine in Everyday Life, edited by Shirley Linden-baum and Margaret Lock. Berkeley: University of California Press (1993): 330–363.

Love, Susan. *Dr. Susan Love's Hormone Book: Making Informed Choices About Menopause*. New York: Random House, 1997.

Lucas, Michel. "Ethyl-Eicosapentaenoic Acid for the Treatment of Psychological Distress and Depressive Symptoms in Middle-Aged Women: A Double-Blind, Placebo-Controlled, Randomized Clinical Trial." *American Journal of Clinical Nutrition* 89 (2) (Feb 2009): 641–651.

Mahady, Gail B., Locklear, Tracie D., et al. "Menopause, A Universal Female Experience: Lessons from Mexico and Central America." *Current Women's Health Reviews* 4 (1) (2008): 3–8.

Manne, Joy. *Conscious Breathing: How Shamanic Breathing Can Change Your Life*. Berkeley, CA: North Atlantic Books, 2004.

Martin, Emily. *The Woman in the Body: A Cultural Analysis of Reproduction*. Boston, MA: Beacon Press, 1987.

Mathias, J. R., et al. "Relation of Endometriosis and Neuromuscular Disease of the Gastrointestinal Tract: New Insights." *Fertility and Sterility* 70 (1) (July 1998): 81–88.

McKinney, C. H., et al. "Effects of Guided Imagery and Music (GIM) Therapy on Mood and Cortisol in Healthy Adults." *Health Psychology* (4) (July 1997): 390–400.

Mead, Margaret. *Coming of Age in Samoa: A Psychological Study of Primitive Youth for Western Civilisation*. New York: Morrow Quill Paperbacks, 1961.

Meadows, Elaine. "Treatments for Patients with Pelvic Pain." *Urologic Nursing* 19 (1) (March 1999): 33–35.

Mongan, Marie F. *Hypnobirthing: A Celebration of Life*. Concord, NH: Rivertree Publishing, 1998.

Morse, C. A., et al. "A Comparison of Hormone Therapy, Coping Skills Training, and Relaxation for the Relief of Premenstrual Syndrome." *Journal of Behavioral Medicine* 14 (5) (1991): 469–489.

Myss, Caroline. *Anatomy of the Spirit: The Seven Stages of Power and Healing*. New York: Three Rivers Press, 1996.

Naparstek, Belleruth. *Staying Well with Guided Imagery*. New York: Warner Books, 1994.

Northrup, Christiane. *Women's Bodies, Women's Wisdom: Creating Physical and Emotional Health and Healing*. New York: Bantam Books, 2006.

Ockene, J. K., et al. "Symptom Experience After Discontinuing Use of Estrogen Plus Progestin." *Journal of the American Medical Association* 294 (2) (July 2005): 183–193.

O'Connell, E. "Mood, Energy, Cognition, and Physical Complaints: A Mind/ Body Approach to Symptom Management During the Climacteric." *Journal of Obstetric, Gynecologic, and Neonatal Nursing* 34 (2) (2005): 274–279.

Parazzini, F., et al. "Selected Food Intake and Risk of Endometriosis." *Human Reproduction* 19 (8) (July 2004): 1755–1759.

Parker, William H., Broder, Michael S., Liu, Zhimei, Shoupe, Donna, et al. "Ovarian Conservation at the Time of Hysterectomy for Benign Disease." *Obstetrics & Gynecology* 106 (2) (August 2005): 219–226.

Pert, Candace B. *The Molecules of Emotion: The Science Behind Mind-Body Medicine.* New York: Touchstone, 1997.

Plourde, Elizabeth. *Hysterectomy and Ovary Removal: What All Women Need to Know.* Irvine, CA: New Voice Publications, 2001.

Pollan, Michael. *The Omnivore's Dilemma: A Natural History of Four Meals.* New York: Penguin Books, 2006.

Profit, Margie. "The Quarterly Review of Biology: Menstruation As a Defense Against Pathogens Transported by Sperm." *The Quarterly Review of Biology* 68 (3) (Sept 1993): 335–381.

Rasmussen, S. J. "From Childbearers to Culture-Bearers: Transition to Postchild-bearing Among Tuareg Women." *Medical Anthropology* 19 (1) (Jul 2000): 91–116.

Redmond, Layne. *When the Drummers Were Women: A Spiritual History of Rhythm.* New York: Three Rivers Press, 1997.

Rees, Barbara. "Effect of Relaxation with Guided Imagery on Anxiety, Depression, and Self-Esteem in Primiparas." *Journal of Holistic Nursing* 13 (3) (1995): 255–267.

Rier, S. E., Martin, D. C., Bowman, R. E., et al. "Endometriosis in Rhesus Monkeys (Maccaca Mulatta) Following Chronic Exposure to 2,3, 7,8-Tetrachlorodibenzo-p-dioxin." *Fundamental and Applied Toxicology* 21 (1993): 433–441.

Rossi, Edoardo. "Fish Oil Derivatives As a Prophylaxis of Recurrent Miscarriage Associated with Antiphospholipid Antibodies (APL): A Pilot Study." *Lupus* 2 (5) (1993): 319–323.

Rossignol, A. M., and Bonnlander, H. "Caffeine-Containing Beverages, Total Fluid Consumption, and Premenstrual Syndrome." *American Journal of Public Health* 80 (9) (1990): 1106–1110.

Rossman, Martin. *Guided Imagery for Self-Healing: An Essential Resource for Anyone Seeking Wellness.* Novato, CA: New World Library, 2000.

Roughead, Zamzam K., Hunt, Janet R., et al. "Controlled Substitution of Soy Protein for Meat Protein: Effects on Calcium Retention, Bone, and Cardio-vascular Health Indices in Postmenopausal Women." *Journal of Clinical Endocrinology & Metabolism* 90 (1) (January 2005): 181–189.

Ruiz, Don Miguel. *The Four Agreements: A Practical Guide to Personal Freedom.* San Rafael, CA: Amber-Allen Publishing, 1997.

Sahin, K., et al. "Lycopene Supplementation Prevents the Development of Spontaneous Smooth Muscle Tumors on the Oviduct in Japanese Quail." *Nutrition and Cancer* 50 (2) (2004): 181–189.

Salvesen, Kjell, and Morkved, Siv. "Randomised Controlled Trial of Pelvic Floor Muscle Training During Pregnancy." *British Journal of Medicine* (329) (July 2004): 378–380.

Sandyk, Reuven, Anastasiadis, P. G., Anninos, P. A., and Tsagas, N. "Is Postmeno-pausal Osteoporosis Related to Pineal Gland Functions?" *International Journal of Neuroscience* 62 (3–4) (1991): 215–225.

Schulte, Christa. *Tantric Sex for Women: A Guide for Lesbian, Bi, Hetero, and Solo Lovers.* Berlin, Germany: Krug and Schadenberg, 2005.

Scott, Pauline. *Sit Up and Take Notice: Positioning Yourself for a Better Birth.* Taranga, New Zealand: Great Scott Publications, 2003.

Shelton, J. D. "Prostacyclin from the Uterus and Woman's Cardiovascular Advantage." *Prostaglandins Leukotrienes and Medicine* 8 (5) (May 1982): 459–466.

Shepperson-Mills, Dian, and Vernon, Michael. *Endometrosis: A Key to Healing Through Nutrition.* London: Thorsons, 2002.

Sherwood, R. A., Rocks, B. F., Stewart, A., and Saxton, R. S. "Magnesium and the Premenstrual Syndrome." *Annals of Clinical Biochemistry* 23 (6) (1986): 667–670.

Shlain, Leonard. *Sex, Time and Power: How Women's Sexuality Shaped Human Evolution.* New York: Penguin, 2003.

Sigmon, S. T., and Nelson, R. O. "The Effectiveness of Activity Scheduling and Relaxation Training in the Treatment of Spasmodic Dysmenorrhea." *Journal of Behavioral Medicine* 11 (5) (1988): 483–495.

Skultans, Vieda. "The Symbolic Significance of Menstruation and the Meno-pause." *Man* 5 (4) (1970): 639–651.

Some, Patrice Malidoma. *Of Water and the Spirit: Ritual, Magic, and Initiation in the Life of an African Shaman.* New York: Arkana, 1994.

Steege, J. F., and Blumenthal, J. A., "The Effects of Aerobic Exercise on Premenstrual Symptoms in Middle-Aged Women: A Preliminary Study." *Journal of Psychosomatic Research* 37 (2) (1993): 127–133.

Strausz, Ivan. *You Don't Need a Hysterectomy: New and Effective Ways of Avoiding Major Surgery*. Reading, MA: Addison-Wesley, 1993.

Sundahl, Deborah. *Female Ejaculation and the G-Spot: Not Your Mother's Orgasm Book*. Alameda, CA: Hunter House, 2003.

Taylor, A. S., Ang, C., Bell, S. C., and Konje, J. C. "The Role of the Endocannabinoid System in Gametogenesis, Implantation, and Early Pregnancy." *Human Reproduction Update* 13 (5) (June 2007): 501–513.

Taylor, Mary, et al. "Participant Perspective on a Yoga Intervention for Menopausal Symptoms." *Complementary Health Practice Review* 13 (3) (2008): 171–181.

Teoman, N., Ozcan, A., and Acar, B. "The Effect of Exercise on Physical Fitness and Quality of Life in Postmenopausal Women." *Maturitas* 47 (1) (2004): 71–77.

Thompson, Lilian. "Dietary Flaxseed Alters Tumor Biological Markers in Postmenopausal Breast Cancer." *Clinical Cancer Research* 11 (May 2005): 3828–3835.

Thorpe, Donna, et al. "Effects of Meat Consumption and Vegetarian Diet on Risk of Wrist Fracture over 25 Years in a Cohort of Peri- and Postmenopausal Women." *Public Health Nutrition* 11 (2008): 564–572.

Thys-Jacobs, Susan. "Micronutrients and the Premenstrual Syndrome: The Case for Calcium." *Journal of the American College of Nutrition* 19 (2) (2000): 220–227.

Thys-Jacobs, Susan, McMahon, Don, and Belezikian, John. "Cyclical Changes in Calcium Metabolism Across the Menstrual Cycle in Women with Premenstrual Dysphoric Disorder." *Journal of Clinical Endocrinology & Metabolism* 92 (8) (2007): 2952–2959.

Tolle, Eckhart. *The Power of Now: A Guide to Spiritual Enlightenment*. Vancouver: Namaste Publishing, 1999.

Turnbull, Colin. *The Forest People*. New York: Simon and Schuster, 1968.

Van de Graaff, Kent M., and Fox, Stuart Ira. *Concepts of Human Anatomy and Physiology*. Dubuque, IA: William C. Brown, 1995.

Walker, Barbara. *The Women's Encyclopedia of Myths and Secrets*. San Francisco, CA: Harper & Row, 1983.

Walker, Morton. *Sexual Nutrition: How to Nutritionally Improve, Enhance, and Stimulate Your Sexual Appetite*. Garden City Park, NY: Avery Publishing Group, 1979.

Wallach, Edward E., and Eisenberg, Esther. *Hysterectomy: Exploring Your Options.* Baltimore, MD: The Johns Hopkins University Press, 2003.

Walsh, Maxwell, and Polus, Barbara. "A Randomized, Placebo-Controlled Clinical Trial on the Efficacy of Chiropractic Therapy on Premenstrual Syndrome." *Journal of Manipulative and Physiological Therapeutics* 22 (9) (1999): 582–585.

Weed, Susun. *Menopausal Years: The Wise Woman Way.* Woodstock, NY: Ash Tree Publishing, 1992.

Weidegger, P. *Menstruation and Menopause: The Physiology and Psychology, the Myth and the Reality.* New York: Alfred A. Knopf, 1976.

Williamson, J., White, A., Hart, A., and Ernst, E. "Randomised Controlled Trial of Reflexology for Menopausal Symptoms." *BJOG—An International Journal of Obstetrics and Gynaecology* 109 (9) (2002): 1050–1055.

Wurn, B. F., et al. "Treating Female Infertility and Improving IVF Pregnancy Rates with a Manual Physical Therapy Technique." *Medscape General Medicine* 6 (2) (June 2004): 51–68.

Wurn, L. J., et al. "Treating Endometriosis Pain with a Manual Pelvic Physical Therapy." *Fertility and Sterility* 86 (3) (Sept 2006): S29–S30.

Young, Serenity. *An Anthology of Sacred Texts By and About Women.* New York: Crossroads Press, 1993.

Zaborowska, E., et al. "Effects of Acupuncture, Applied Relaxation, Estrogens and Placebo on Hot Flushes in Postmenopausal Women: An Analysis of Two Prospective, Parallel, Randomized Studies." *Climacteric* 10 (1) (June 2007): 38–45.

Zondervan, K. T., et al. "Oral Contraceptives and Cervical Cancer—Further Findings from the Oxford Family Planning Association Contraceptive Study." *British Journal of Cancer* 73 (10) (May 1996): 1291–1297.

Index

Printed in the United States
by Baker & Taylor Publisher Services